Medical Ethics,
Human Choices

Medical Ethics, Human Choices

A CHRISTIAN PERSPECTIVE

Edited by

John Rogers

HERALD PRESS
Scottdale, Pennsylvania
Kitchener, Ontario

Library of Congress Cataloging-in-Publication Data

Medical ethics, human choices.

Bibliography: p.
1. Medical ethics. 2. Medicine—Religious aspects—
Christianity. I. Rogers, John, 1951-
R725.56.M44   1988   241'.642   87-29747
ISBN 0-8361-3460-5 (pbk.)

241.6
M

Scripture taken from the *Holy Bible: New International Version,* copyright © 1973, 1978, 1984 by the International Bible Society. Used by permission of Zondervan Bible Publishers.

Contents

Increased technical capacity has forced us to face new ethical-moral questions related to medical-health care. Does can do *mean* should do—*and for whom?*

We cannot understand what kind of moral character we ought to nourish within our communities and what kinds of behavior are appropriate for us as Christians without some understanding of what kind of creatures we are, having been made "in the image of God."

The church should avoid simple, short-sighted solutions to present medical crises. With the medical community, it has a responsibility to recognize and accept the emerging challenges and opportunities.

Foreword

LeRoy Walters

Center for Bioethics, Kennedy Institute of Ethics,
Georgetown University, Washington, D.C.

Medical ethics has become a laypeople's movement of the 1970s
and 1980s. New medical technologies—respirators, kidney dialysis,
and heart transplantation—helped to spark the movement. But
social upheavals of the 1960s also contributed to the extension of
this field beyond medical professionals. It is no accident that
popular concern around medical ethics developed close on the heels
of popular involvement in the Civil Rights Movement and anti-
Vietnam War protests. Traditional structures of authority were being called into question in numerous social spheres.

Before laypeople became deeply involved in medical ethics,
there had been two major kinds of professional literature in this
area. Health professionals, usually physicians or nurses, had
developed codes of ethics and had written articles for their own
colleagues in professional journals. Within the Christian church,
Catholic and Anglican moral theologians had produced textbooks
of medical ethics directed toward the clergy on the one hand and
toward health professionals on the other (LeRoy Walters, "Medical
Ethics," *New Catholic Encyclopedia: Supplement, 1967-74* [New
York: McGraw-Hill, 1974], pp. 290-91). What was lacking in traditional medical ethics was the sense that the perspective of the

patient and layperson is essential to well-rounded ethical discussion.

All of that has changed. Many books and articles on medical ethics directed toward laypeople are now available. These works have been written by people trained in a startling variety of disciplines, including theology, philosophy, and literature. Courses in medical ethics are offered to undergraduate majors in every field, as well as to continuing-education students in numerous professions. In some states and local communities, citizens have initiated grassroots efforts to discuss medical ethics questions. Oregon Health Decisions, the prototype for such initiatives, culminated in a statewide health parliament (Ralph Crawshaw, et al., "Oregon Health Decisions: An Experiment with Informed Community Consent," *Journal of the American Medical Association* 254 [13 December 1985]: 3213-16).

In a most interesting and original way, this book demonstrates that medical ethics has become a laypeople's movement. The content was decisively shaped by discussions with a cross-section of members from local congregations. The book is now being returned to the local congregations as a resource for discussion, for familial decision making, and perhaps for community action. Careful readers will note that it covers both micro-level and macro-level problems. Decisions about appropriate treatment for a critically ill parent usually involve only a few family members and one or two health professionals. In contrast, programs of health promotion and long-term planning for hospital construction and health insurance coverage are system-level issues. Micro-level problems are immediate and vivid. We all have faced them and will face them again. Health system problems are more unclear and sometimes more threatening. But timely involvement at the system (macro-) level by congregations can help to ensure that more humane alternatives are available when micro-level decisions confront us.

This book is a pioneering effort to respond to the expressed concerns of local congregations and to a new array of biomedical possibilities. In a very real sense it challenges us to expand the scope of the Christian love ethic. This creative work illustrates how members of the local community of caring Christians can incorporate a new dimension into their thinking, their mutual support, and their outreach to the larger society.

Preface

John Rogers

In the accounts of the first human sin from Genesis 3 and 4, two significant commonalities are central to the theme of this book. First, when confronted with their transgressions, Adam, Eve, and Cain all try to become irresponsible. God looks for Adam and Eve after they have eaten from the forbidden tree. When God discovers their sin, their response is to make excuses for their choices. Adam even tries to distance himself from his spouse. When God confronts Cain about the absence of his brother, Abel, Cain tries to evade God's probing. He asks whether he is responsible for his brother's welfare.

Second, however, in each case God does not allow the persons to be irresponsible. God calls them to task for what they have done and forces them to bear the weight of their choices. This is not simply judgment; it is grace. God calls them to continue to exercise the authority and to live in the community that God has given them. To allow them to be irresponsible would run counter to God's original investment in them. To let them arbitrarily separate themselves would have put them in a state of isolation, which God had already declared as not good.

Having been made to live in the image of God, we are called to exercise authority. This also means that we are called to be responsible and accountable for who we are and what we do—individually and collectively. In the absence of these qualities—authority, responsibility, accountability, and community, or solidarity—we likely will not realize the potential of our humanness, of our having been created to live in the image of God.

The aim of this book, *Medical Ethics, Human Choices*, is to assist the reader in reaffirming the fundamental authority and consequent responsibility that are ours in relation to medical dilemmas and crises. In a time of increasing technical capacity it is easy to lose sight of these essential qualities of being human. In the area of medicine and health care, we may be tempted to look for simple technical answers to complex and fundamentally human questions.

The issues that surround medical dilemmas and crises are, at root, questions of human authority, responsibility, and solidarity. The bottom line for the Christian is this: How will I live "in the image of God" in the face of these dilemmas and crises? How will I be critically and creatively loving in the presence of pain and suffering and possibly death? This is not a simplistic attempt to reduce the tension that accompanies stressful medical situations. Rather, it is an attempt to bring to bear on them the full resources of our being—body, mind, spirit—individually and communally.

The cover of this book suggests that we hold the mystery of life in our hands. We are stewards of life itself. Behind the medical jargon and paraphernalia human hearts are at work—hearts of perception, perspective, valuing, hope, inspiration, commitment. The choices that emerge impact not only the persons under consideration, but also those whom they will touch in various ways. Solidarity is part of our having been made to live in the image of God. Thus we are called to responsible, critical, creative—which is to say loving—communion with the medical communities that can assist us in living into the image of God. The goal of this book is to help that communion to take place.

This brings me back to the Genesis stories that I referred to initially. Adam, Eve, and Cain also held the mystery of life in their hands. In that sense, they had authority. They were entrusted with authority. And they became responsible and accountable. They could not become irresponsible, even though they tried.

We too cannot become irresponsible. That is, we cannot give

up our responsibility as stewards of life. We can only choose how to exercise our stewardship. For us who have embraced the Christian story and vision, faithful stewardship includes loving God with our whole being and loving our neighbors as ourselves. Our funda-mental Christian vocation, or calling, is to be unique expressions of that love. This love ultimately comes from God. I hope this book will help you to make this principle of Christian faith concrete when facing medical dilemmas and crises. For we are each other's keepers.

Acknowledgments

In 1985 Mennonite Mutual Aid (MMA), Goshen, Indiana, called together a Health Ethics Review Committee to help it and its constituents consider appropriate responses to the ever-rising river of ethical dilemmas we are facing in relation to medical care. Included in the committee were representatives of the health and legal professions, educators, ethicists, and congregational leaders: Bob Cain, administrator of the Brethren Home, Greenville, Ohio; LeRoy Friesen, professor of peace studies, Associated Mennonite Biblical Seminaries, Elkhart, Indiana; Anne Krabill Hershberger, associate professor of nursing at Goshen College, Goshen, Indiana; Ron Ropp, vice-president of the Illinois Pastoral Services Institute, Bloomington, Illinois; Evelyn Rouner, retired college professor in family/child studies, from Colwich Kansas; Bob Shreiner, pastor at Hyattsville Mennonite Church, Hyattsville, Maryland; Carol Suter, an attorney from Bluffton, Ohio; and Marjorie Gerbrandt Wiens, a cardiologist from Fresno, California. Consultants for this group were Willard Krabill, physician for Goshen College; and LeRoy Walters, director of the Center for Bioethics of the Kennedy Institute of Ethics, Georgetown University, Washington, D.C.

The committee recommended initially that MMA hold "hearings" in various population centers of Mennonite and Brethren churches. MMA accepted this suggestion and held these hearings in Harrisonburg, Virginia; Newton, Kansas; Fresno, California; Blooming Glen, Pennsylvania; Strasburg, Pennsylvania; Goshen, Indiana; and Louisville, Ohio.

At each of the hearings there were stories of pain in dealing with the intimidating health care system; stories of tough decisions that had to be made—and no one to help make them; stories that questioned whether the right decision had been made in discontinuing, or continuing, life-prolonging treatment. At one hearing was a man who had been in a coma for many months, on whom life support systems were discontinued, but who then experienced an amazing degree of recovery. At another hearing was a husband and father who two weeks before had buried his wife who had been in a profound coma for over three years. At another was a person who had been rejected for a heart-lung transplant.

The committee quickly recognized the need for churches to examine together and reach consensus on some crucial questions. What is the Christian witness on the use of today's expensive medical technology? What is the role of the congregation in helping its members deal with tragic choices? So they recommended that MMA work with the Mennonite Publishing House to produce a study guide to help congregations work with the difficult questions that we must face in relation to medical technology. Again, MMA accepted this suggestion and called together a reference group to plan the study guide: Willard Krabill, physician; Tana Durnbaugh, health educator-administrator; Beverly Holmskog, congregational leader and educator; and Clarence Rempel, pastor.

Assisting the Health Ethics Review Committee and the planning group for the study guide were staff Ron Litwiller, then Mutual Aid Services vice-president; Charlotte Schrag Sprunger and Darlene Hochstetler, MMA support staff; and Helen Alderfer, coordinator for the study guide project.

It is the prayer of all of who have had a part in the development of this book that it will be a significant instrument in our common quest for greater faithfulness to God and the church of Jesus Christ—particularly when facing difficult medical decisions.

Contributors

CONRAD G. BRUNK (Chapter 2) is associate professor of philosophy and Peace and Conflict Studies at Conrad Grebel College, Waterloo, Ontario.

TANA DURNBAUGH (Chapter 6) is director of the Center for Health Professional Continuing Education, College of Lake County, Grayslake, Illinois.

MYRON EBERSOLE (Chapter 9) is director of Pastoral Services at the Milton S. Hershey Medical Center, Hershey, Pennsylvania.

STAN GODSHALL (Chapter 11) is a family physician at the Norlanco Family Health Center, Elizabethtown, Pennsylvania.

ANNE KRABILL HERSHBERGER (Chapter 8) is associate professor of nursing at Goshen College, Goshen, Indiana.

PAUL W. HOFFMAN (Chapter 10) is president and professor of psychology at McPherson College, McPherson, Kansas.

WILLARD S. KRABILL (Chapters 1 and 4) is the physician for Goshen College, Goshen, Indiana, where he also teaches courses in human sexuality and substance abuse.

HOWARD J. LOEWEN (Chapter 3) is associate professor of theology at Mennonite Brethren Biblical Seminary, Fresno, California.

ANN RABER (Chapter 12) is director of the Wellness Program of Mennonite Mutual Aid, Goshen, Indiana.

JOHN ROGERS is an editor in the Congregational Literature Division of the Mennonite Publishing House.

DAVID SCHROEDER (Chapter 5) is professor of New Testament and philosophy at Canadian Mennonite Bible College, Winnipeg, Manitoba.

ERLAND WALTNER (Chapter 13) is professor of English Bible at the Associated Mennonite Biblical Seminaries, Elkhart, Indiana, and executive secretary of the Mennonite Medical Association.

JESSE H. ZIEGLER (Chapter 7) is professor of Medicine in Society in the School of Medicine at Wright State University, Dayton, Ohio.

Medical Ethics,
Human Choices

1

Medical Ethics: Facing Difficult Questions

Willard S. Krabill

SEVERAL YEARS AGO, a young woman came to the office of the director of Mutual Aid Services at Mennonite Mutual Aid Association in Goshen, Indiana. "I don't know whether to thank you or scold you," she said. Since he had never met her before, Ron Litwiller was taken aback. She then told Ron about her niece, an infant born with severe multiple handicaps and disabilities. It was clear from the start that she could never be a normal functioning human being. Indeed, it was clear that she was unlikely to survive a year. Over the next eight months until her death, MMA spent $100,000 of its members' premium dollars in the care of this infant, a futile cause.

"Some would have called her a vegetable," the aunt continued. "But, I knew she was not a vegetable, a carrot. I held her. She was a human being. We loved her. I appreciate what MMA did for her and for our family. But, really, is it justifiable to spend that much money in an effort that we knew from the start was futile?"

Defining Terms

Ethics can be a complex philosophical study. But what we are really talking about here are the *shoulds* and *oughts* of life. We are talking about the right principles by which we make decisions.

When grandmother is wasting away, unable to speak, walk, eat, or recognize anyone, what principles should guide us? How do we decide whether to give her antibiotics for her pneumonia or to force-feed her with a tube through her nose?

Perhaps you have heard the term *medical ethics* before. Maybe you thought of it as the proper action of doctors and nurses. In this book, we will use the term to cover that and more. For now, think of medical ethics as including the shoulds and oughts that all of us face in our dealings with issues in our medical-health care and with all aspects of the health care system.

Health care is another confusing term. What we usually call health care is really sickness care, or medical care. Americans spend over a billion dollars a day on sickness care. If we had a health care system with a proper emphasis on keeping healthy, we wouldn't have to spend so much. Nevertheless, popular use of the term *health care* includes everything related to medicine: medical care, physical health, drugs, treatment, rehabilitation, and more.

We should also define what we mean by *ethical dilemmas* in relation to medical-health care. A dilemma is a situation requiring a choice between at least two alternatives that are equally compelling and for which we can make equally strong cases. Modern medical technology has created many situations in which there is no simple right or wrong answer. If a common-sense answer is available, it is not a dilemma. If a parent decides not to call a physician to care for a diabetic teenager, a part of us responds that adults should not be allowed to jeopardize the welfare of their minor children. But another part of us is aware of the rights and prerogatives of parents, the need for ordered family life, and the freedom of religious expression. That part responds that no one should interfere in a family's religious practice. That illustrates a dilemma.

Maybe there was a time when right was right, wrong was wrong, and that was that. When it comes to decisions in health care, that time is past. Modern medicine presents us with true dilemmas. It may be impossible to both relieve pain and prolong life, impossible to both opt for a heart transplant and be a good neighbor in the world community, impossible to save my handicapped child's life and at the same time provide my other children with adequate parenting and an education.

Since the late 1960s, our society has been moving further toward affirming the right of the individual to decide about medical care (the ethical principle of *autonomy*). In 1982, the President's Commission for the Study of Ethical Problems in Medicine stated that the competent adult, or his or her properly chosen surrogate, has the right to decline medical treatment even though that would result in death.

We are living in an era of rights—especially individual rights. This fact presents physicians with another ethical dilemma. Physicians are committed to do what is best for the patient (the ethical principles of *beneficence* and *doing no harm*). What, then, should physicians do when the best course of medical treatment seems clear, but the patient rejects the advice—especially if he says, "I prefer to die"? When the principles of autonomy and beneficence collide, which should prevail? To what extent is the physician justified in manipulating the information given to patients to gain acceptance of what is best for them from the physician's standpoint?

How Did We Get Where We Are Today?

In the remainder of this chapter, we will look at what happened to make medical ethics such an important concern in a relatively short time. We also will ask why we need to try to reach some agreements or consensus in the church about the shoulds and oughts that will guide us in choosing not only a Christian lifestyle but also a Christian death style. Finally, we will consider why medical ethics should be a major concern for Christians.

Many streams have converged to create the river of ethical dilemmas we face in medical-health care. The most noticeable, and perhaps the most forceful, is the rapid advance of medical technology in the past thirty-five years. Phenomenal techniques and equipment have been devised for the treatment of illness. Some of them have been obviously helpful, others not so helpful. But most have given rise to serious ethical questions as to the appropriate use of expensive technology. The concern is especially troublesome in the care of persons whose lives are spent—particularly when we consider the needs of our brothers and sisters in the third world who don't have the resources to immunize their children or to assure a safe water supply.

We hear of brain-dead pregnant women being kept "alive" until the fetus is old enough to deliver by cesarean section. We hear of the newborn with five parents: the woman who donated the egg, the man who donated the sperm, the woman who rented her uterus, and the couple who then raise the child. Medical technology has given most of us the ability to influence the time and manner of our dying. And over 10 percent of us will directly confront the issue of withholding or withdrawing life-sustaining treatment. Medical research has devised feeding formulas that enable tube-fed individuals to be maintained indefinitely. It is all very marvelous, fantastic—technologically.

But what about the emotional, financial, spiritual, and humanitarian dimensions? These are the ethical questions, deeply personal questions. All of us will face them sooner or later. The dilemma is captured in what has come to be known as "the technological imperative." Does the fact that the technology exists mean that we have to use it always? Does *can do* mean *should do*?

Another stream that contributes to our river of dilemmas is today's economic climate. Medical costs have grown at such a tremendous rate that cutting those costs has become a major goal of businesses, government, insurance companies, and families. In the process, providing health care has become a business in which financial considerations often outweigh human need. However, there is competition for dollars in our society. In its love affair with technology, we tend to pay for the research and the machines. But we raise Medicare deductibles, cut medical benefits for the poor, and close neighborhood health centers. Two years ago, the California legislature voted to pay for heart transplants and a week later dropped 250,000 poor people from Medicaid coverage. We already *can do* more than we are willing to pay for—more than we are willing to make available to all. Thus, the further expansion of medical technological capability only widens the gap between what we can do and what we will do.

Justice in medical-health care is another serious ethical issue. By the way we use medical services and technology, we Christians make a statement regarding our beliefs about life, suffering, death, and justice. Can we agree what that statement should be?

Other streams converge to increase the dilemmas we face. For example, we do not emphasize prevention, including prevention of birth defects. It makes much more sense to reduce the number of low birth-weight newborns than to spend the millions we do on neonatal intensive care units. There is also the stream of the graying of America. The numbers of the elderly are moving rapidly from 12 percent to 18 or 20 percent of the population. The increased mobility of our society results in weakening the stability of home and family. The care of the disabled elderly was once a family responsibility. It is now a public responsibility. Our society has become "medicalized" as we apply the medical or disease models to more and more of society's ills. This has led to unrealistic expectations of what medicine can deliver. We are a society in which lawsuits are seen as the way to right all wrongs. The result has been a drastic increase in the cost of medical care and medical products. All of these streams converge to create a river of dilemmas that affect all of us.

A Christian Concern

The study of the shoulds and oughts surrounding the use of our bodies and of health care resources is at the intersection of our faith and our health behavior. At stake is what we believe it means to be in the image of God. In the process of being born or in the process of dying, when are we no longer in God's image? What and when is death? Are personal death and biological death the same? Do they occur at the same time?

In making decisions about our health care, we are confronted by an intimidating medical system whose professionals usually operate under the assumption that this is a biological world. Reality consists of gene structures, molecules, and cells; and medical science eventually will explain all human biological phenomena. When the focus is on the physical to the exclusion of the spiritual—when the focus is exclusively on beating hearts and breathing lungs—then it is quite normal to cling tenaciously to biological existence.

The world around us looks at these ethical dilemmas in a secular way. It is as if the issues are political, social, and economic— matters of public policy. They are these, but they are more. The issues are profoundly and basically religious. If we allow the assumptions or prescriptions of the system to dictate our decisions, we will err badly and do violence to our Christian faith and witness. The divorce of science and faith is the source of many of the dilemmas that we face. In our witness to the world, the study of medical ethics is a Christian concern.

The church should provide a climate, an environment, where brothers and sisters can face difficult choices together. Rather than arriving at isolated or individualistic decisions, we can make decisions in concert with brothers and sisters in our family of faith. We also need to provide support for those who have already made difficult decisions and wonder if they made the right choice. To make these kinds of decisions is a lonely experience. We need to support those who have made them and help alleviate the sense of doubt and guilt that often accompanies them. Over and over I hear the question, "Did we do the right thing?"

We need to encourage and support each other as we attempt to deal with an impersonal health care system. We need to realize the evangelistic potential of our loving and caring. The way we help each other and the way that we acknowledge our dependence on each other is contagious and enhances our evangelistic outreach.

These ethical issues are a Christian concern because our society is unjust in its health care for the poor. Neighborhood health centers are closing, Medicare deductibles are rising, Medicaid rolls are being cut back, access to health care by poor people is more difficult, and the numbers of people in the U.S. with inadequate or no health insurance has risen to 35 million. Ability to pay certainly *is* a factor in the level of services available. And this injustice is further compounded by the disparity between what is available in North America as compared to brothers and sisters in developing countries.

Ethicist Stanley Hauerwas asks whether Christian people are at the point where they are ready to say, "Even though I have the resources, or even if I have the insurance coverage to make it possible, I will rather forgo the utilization of expensive life-extending technology so that others might have basic care which my utilization of expensive resources might deny them." In a similar vein, Daniel Conrad, a Mennonite physician, suggests that

> presently we are approaching the sensitive questions very gingerly by asking, "Is it ever right *not to expend* all available resources to save

life?" I would like to suggest that a better question for the rich Christian community confronted with a Lazarus-world population might be, "Is it ever right *to expend* all available resources?" I hope that as more sensitivity to these issues develops on the part of "care consumers," there will develop a body of conscientious objectors and even health care resisters in our [church] community.

In our congregations, we also should address the issue of how we want our insurance companies to spend our medical and health-premium dollars—on what technology, on the maintenance of what degree of "life"—keeping in mind our overall mission as the church, not only in this country but around the world. We are bound to each other in mutual aid. This is another important reason these matters are a Christian concern.

For Discussion

1. What pain have members of your congregation experienced in facing medical dilemmas? Was the congregation involved and helpful?

2. When did you first become aware of ethical questions in relation to medical-health care?

3. How did you react when you heard about the artificial heart? About Baby Jesse and the baboon heart?

4. Have you visited some of the "worse-off" people in your local nursing home?

5. If you were Karen Quinlan's parents, would you have continued to tube-feed her for ten years?

6. Considering our concern for mission and service around the world to what extent should medical insurance premiums be used to pay for very expensive high-tech medical and surgical procedures—such as heart-lung transplants?

7. Is it ever right to spend all we can to prolong someone's life?

8. Do you carry an organ donor card in your billfold? Why or why not?

9. Has this chapter helped motivate you to live a healthier prevention-oriented lifestyle? What practical steps might you begin with?

10. How can we work toward consensus in the congregation about the proper expenditure of money for health care when our incomes and our medical needs are so different?

2

In the Image of God

Conrad G. Brunk

NO CHRISTIAN APPROACH to medical ethics can hope to get very far without coming to terms with what it means to be a person. This is true because the concept of personhood is at the center of Christian ethics. We cannot fully understand what is good or evil, what kind of moral character we ought to nourish within our communities, and what kinds of behavior are appropriate for us as Christians without some understanding of what kind of creatures we are.

Modern philosophical theories of ethics generally are skeptical of our ability to observe any kind of *human nature* from which we can deduce what is *natural* and therefore good for men and women. Many Christian theologians, especially the Protestant Reformers and the Anabaptists, also doubted this possibility. They believed that whatever God may have created Adam and Eve to be, the perversion of human nature by sin erased the last vestiges of natural goodness with which they were created.

These philosophers and theologians may be right. But even if they are, it does not mean that no such thing as human nature exists. It means only that our knowledge of it cannot be obtained from observation of the way men and women actually live. Rather, it is obtainable only from what God has revealed to us in the Scriptures and in Jesus.

As Christians we believe that we are *creatures*, that we have been made by a Creator whose purposes transcend our own desires. We also believe that we have been created *in the very image of God* and that regardless of how this image has been corrupted by sin, it still represents the standard of humanness as it should be. This belief in God's own image within us—this spark of the divine nature itself which sets us apart from all other creatures—is central to all discussions about what kind of people we ought to be. It is at the core of what we mean when we speak of the Christian view of *person*.

The idea that we are simply sentient beings—beings capable of experiencing pleasures and pains, happiness and misery, in much the same way as lower animals, only with greater discrimination—dominates much of the contemporary, secular discussion of morality in medicine. In this view, we measure goodness only in terms of how much pleasure or happiness can be brought about in the world. Evil is measured in terms of how much pain or misery is to be avoided by our actions. The value of our existence lies only in the experiences we have. There is no value inherent in each of us, regardless of the quality of the experiences we happen to have. Life has value only if its pleasures outweigh its pains. It has no purpose or value beyond itself.

In this view, then, there is no moral problem in aborting fetuses with unwanted characteristics or the "mercy killing" of oneself (suicide) or others (active euthanasia) when life proves to be a burden. Nothing other than the sum total of pleasures and pains in life makes any moral difference.

For Christians, however, there is more to each of us than the quality of our particular experience. There is the intrinsic value of our selves—our unique personhood—which derives from that divine image in which we were molded at our creation. We cannot decide the hard questions of moral right and wrong without taking seriously this intrinsic value.

Personhood and the Image of God

What are the elements of God's image in us which shape our

concept of personhood and our ethical understanding? This is not an easy question to answer. While the Bible is clear that we are created in God's image, it is not always as clear which attributes of God we share. Clearly, we do not share God's omnipotence, omniscience, omnipresence, and perfect goodness. These belong only to God as the absolute source of all being. So we have to look carefully at what the Scriptures tell us about the nature of God and the nature of humanity. We are created "a little lower than the angels," yet a little higher than the lower animals, the Bible tells us. One way to understand the nature of our personhood, then, is to look at those characteristics that distinguish us from other animals.

A fundamental characteristic unique to the human animal and shared with the divine nature is the ability to choose between good and evil. Only persons can be morally responsible. We cannot judge the actions and character of nonhuman animals as morally good or evil, for they are not free to act other than their natures and their circumstances dictate. But we have the ability to transcend in thought and imagination our particular circumstances. This enables us to decide how to act on the basis of what ought to be, rather than merely on the basis of what is. The freedom to choose between good and evil is not only part of our God-likeness; it also is the source of the seemingly limitless evil of which humanity is capable. The Genesis account of the Fall is the story of how the very part of our nature that makes us most like our Creator—knowledge of good and evil—is also the source of the potential undoing of God's will in the world.

Our freedom of will—sometimes called *autonomy*—is possible only because there are other aspects of the image of God that we share. One of the most important of these is our ability to think, or reason—the ability to form concepts that help us to organize our experiences and communicate them to others in language. Again, the Genesis account identifies this unique ability in its reference to God granting to Adam the power to *name* all the other creatures. Only humans have the ability to name what we experience, so that we can think and talk abstractly. Only persons can think and say things that are *true* or *false*. So, only persons can lie and be lied to. Thus, language—the ability to communicate in abstract symbols—is a defining aspect of personhood.

Despite the efforts of scientists to teach some animals the fundamental elements of language in this sense, still only persons have the ability to form an unlimited number of concepts and symbols. This linguistic ability is important, not only because it allows us to think and reason, but also because it illustrates yet another aspect of what it is to be a person—community.

The abilities to think and reason and to exercise free will and act as responsible moral agents all depend upon language. But language can develop only in a community of persons. There can be no such thing as a purely private language—a language that a person could teach oneself and use as the tool for one's own thinking. Thus, to be a person—to have the characteristics of personhood—is to be part of a community. It is to be inextricably linked to others, no matter how isolated or alone we may be at times. Perhaps it is for this reason that even God's own self-reference in Genesis is plural—"Let us make man in our image ... male and female" (Genesis 1:26-27). And perhaps, too, this is the deeper significance of God's observation at the creation of Eve: "It is not good for the man to be alone" (2:18).

Our sense of individual identity—our self-concept—is made possible because we are members of a community. A unique aspect of personhood seems to be that we have a concept of ourselves as unique, individual *selves*. We are aware that we had a beginning and that we shall have an end—death. Lower animals have instinctive fears of pain and threat to their desires, but they cannot fear their own deaths. We humans do this because we are aware of ourselves as individuals who are not the same as the other members of our community.

In this way individuality and community are not opposites of each other. They complement each other. Each requires the other. Thus, in a Christian ethic, respect for individual identity and autonomy is a fundamental value. But we must never isolate individual rights and freedom from the good of the community that nourishes the individual.

Doing what is right and good often requires sacrificing our own desires and interests for the benefit of others. To act morally is to be able to see how our actions affect others and to act for their benefit even when it may not be in our best interest to do so.

The whole of morality is summed up in the ability to "love your neighbor as yourself." Only humans have the capacity to do this. Lower animals act in accord with their appetites and instincts, not in accord with an understanding of what is good for others.

Perhaps this aspect of the human person—the ability to consider unselfishly and unconditionally the needs of others—most importantly reflects the image of God. This is the ability to love in the sense of *agape*—the way in which God loves us. Agape love is not an emotion or a feeling, like those involved in erotic love or in friendship. Rather, it is the ability to serve others for the sake of their own needs. The ability to love is not only at the heart of the Christian concept of the person; it is also the heart of the Christian approach to the moral life.

In summary, the Christian concept of the person as "the image of God" includes the following among its most distinguishing characteristics:

1. The capacity to reason and to communicate in abstract symbols—language.

2. The capacity to have a concept of self as mortal in community with other mortal selves.

3. The capacity for moral autonomy and responsibility.

4. The capacity to subordinate one's own needs and interests to those of others—the capacity to love.

The dangers involved in any attempt to list the aspects of personhood in this way are two. The first is thinking that each characteristic is a necessary condition of personhood. Rather, each is part of a cluster of characteristics that comprise a very complex and mysterious entity—the person. They show us why we can be sure about the clear cases—where all of the characteristics are clearly present or where all or most are absent. But this does not allow us to focus on any one of the characteristics as absolutely essential.

The second danger is to conclude that to be a person, each characteristic must be developed to a high degree. This ignores the fact that most uniquely human attributes need to be nurtured and developed. What defines the person is not development per se, but the *potential* for development. The difference between a chimpanzee and a newborn baby lies in the fact that the chimp lacks the potential to develop any of the characteristics of personhood, while the baby possesses this potential.

Ethical Implications of Personhood

The Christian concept of personhood implies that the dignity and worth of a person has nothing to do with the characteristics that person has through birth or nurture. A person's race, intelligence, attractiveness, health, social status, and even moral character have nothing to do with how much others should value one's life and interests. Our worth lies, not in our accidental attributes or achievements, but solely in the fact that as persons we have the intrinsic worth of God's very image within us.

All persons are of equal dignity and worth. All have an equal claim upon others to the same level of concern for their needs and interests. The right of a seriously genetically impaired newborn to care from its surrounding community is no less than that of any other baby. In a Christian community, decisions regarding its care are not to be based on how much that baby will be able to contribute to our happiness or to the well-being of others. Nor should the decisions be based on how much of a burden its needs will place upon us. The basis for decision-making will be its claim to equal worth as a full member of the community.

This does not mean that we are obligated to spend all of our resources to meet such needs. It means only that whatever we are willing to do for the more attractive baby, we will do for the less attractive. A community that believes in the unconditional and equal worth of persons will view the health care needs of others as a concern of the community simply because they are needs, not because they are one person's needs rather than another's.

The view of persons as being *in the image of God* also means that we make our decisions about who receives care on the basis of what respects the dignity and worth of the persons themselves, not on how it affects others. Philosophers have called this the "respect for persons principle," or the principle that persons should be treated as ends in themselves, not as the means to other persons' ends. So we decide whether to continue or discontinue treatment of the helpless or incompetent, or whether to proceed with an experimental procedure, on the basis of what is in the best interest of the patient, not what is the best interest of others who stand to gain or lose. A decision to "pull the plug" on a life support because it makes the family's life easier violates the dignity of the patient. So too might the decision not to pull the plug if it is motivated by non-patient-centered interests, such as the interest of a physician not to lose a patient.

An agape ethic of unconditional, equal concern for persons demands that in our desire to promote health and other important social goods, we do not use means that undermine personhood and the equal dignity of persons. The implications of this principle for medical ethics are wide ranging. The decision to withhold or distort the truth about patients' conditions denyies them autonomy. The genetic interventions we make in our offspring could potentially undermine their own full personhood. Because God created us *in the divine image*, which includes the ability to build technologies, we have the power to destroy that image in our own children in our attempt to make them "healthier" or "better" in some way.

Personhood and the Sanctity of Life

The view of persons as *in the image of God* has profound implications for several of the most difficult problems in medical ethics. These have to do with the definitions of life and death and the question of how long we should strive to preserve life. When, if ever, abortion is permissible involves the issue of when life begins. Withholding or withdrawing life-saving treatment from the terminally ill involves the issue of when life ends—as well as the question of whether it can be said, from a Christian point of view, that life is no longer the most important value to preserve. Our understanding of personhood and its relation to biological life will influence how we answer these questions.

It is clear, both from the way I have defined personhood and from the way the Bible speaks of life and death, that being a person in the full sense of the word involves more than being a living biological organism. Nothing is clearer in the Christian theological tradition than that the person is more than a material body and that the death of the material body is not identical with the death of the person. Traditionally, this has been put in terms of the distinction between *soul* and *body*. Unlike the Greeks, who also made this distinction, the Christian view is that the person is *both* soul and body. Hence, the apostle Paul's claim that personal life after death requires a resurrected *body*. The important point is that while to be a person is to have a body, certainly the person is more than just a material body or biological organism.

If we admit that there can be organic life—even organic human life—that lacks all the aspects of personhood, then we admit that a living human organism may not be a human person. This is what we do in hospitals when we pronounce people dead while their bodily organs are still functioning. We declare the *person* to be dead because of the evidence that capacity for conscious awareness has been irreversibly lost. I know of no Christians who have protested this so-called "whole-brain death" criterion of the death of a person; nor do I know of any reason why we should. Since the capacity for conscious awareness is necessary for any of the aspects of human personhood to be present, the loss of this capacity provides a solid ground for considering the person no longer alive.

Some Christians would argue that a human embryo or fetus in the very early stages before it develops brain activity is in a similar state. It is a human organism which is *not yet* a person. This was basically the position held by two great theologians of the church, Augustine and Aquinas, who believed that God placed the soul in the body some time after conception. But here the case is less clear, because there is a sense in which the human embryo or fetus has the potential to develop the aspects of personality and the brain-dead person does not. Sincere Christians disagree about the significance of this potential for the personhood of the fetus. It involves very complex issues upon which the Bible sheds little light.

But this leads us to the question of the value of human life itself, regardless of whether it is *personal* human life. Some Christians maintain that even if the early fetus is not a person in the full sense of the term, that it is a developing human life is enough to settle the issue of whether it may ever be aborted. They defend this position on the grounds that human life itself has *absolute sanctity,* or *absolute value*. Those who hold this view also often maintain that we are obligated to go all out to keep even the terminally ill alive as long as possible. But this idea conflicts with other aspects of a biblical, Christian understanding.

Though the Christian view surely affirms the sanctity of the human person as *in the image of God*, this is not the same as the sanctity of the biological life of the person. The Bible does not teach that human life per se is of absolute value. That it is a miraculous gift of God, to be nourished and dedicated with the utmost steward-ship to the service of God and humanity, there can be no doubt. But there is no biblical warrant for unconditionally placing the pres-ervation or prolonging of life above all other values.

The clearest evidence of this is that the Scripture and the whole of Christian tradition hold Christian martyrdom—the deliberate willingness to sacrifice one's own life for one's faith or in the service of others—in the highest esteem. "Greater love has no one than this, that one lay down his life for his friends" (John 15:13). What clearer evidence could we have that Jesus did not consider human life to be absolute in value, nor its maintenance an absolute duty? Jesus points out that life is subordinate to loving concern for the life and interests of *persons*, who have absolute sanctity. The idea that human life itself is higher than all other earthly values and that death is the greatest of all evils is pagan, not Christian. For the Christian, bodily death is not an absolute evil; for death has lost its sting, and the grave its victory.

The teachings of Jesus and the New Testament writers on how to treat one's enemies never appeal to the value or sanctity of life, to say nothing of its *absolute* value or sanctity. Christian nonresistance or nonviolence is based on Jesus' call to his disciples to practice un-conditional love toward their neighbors, whether friend or enemy. Agape love, not the absolute sanctity of life, is the "whole of the law and the prophets." The Christian refusal to take the life of the enemy stems from the law of love, not any absolute value placed upon life itself. Thus, as Jesus says in Matthew 5, "thou shalt not kill" is not enough. We must also love and not hate. This love shows itself, as the whole of Jesus' teachings emphasize, by not pre-ferring our own needs and interests over those of our neighbor.

In short, Jesus shows us that we cannot kill our enemies, be-cause love does not permit us to prefer our own lives and interests to theirs. Christian nonviolence is rooted in the truth that to inflict irreparable injury upon persons, especially taking their lives, is to deny them the equal dignity they enjoy as personal bearers of God's image. Killing is wrong, not primarily because human life itself is sacred, but because the violent destruction of another person's life is among the most grievous harms one person can inflict upon another. The object of agape love, then, is not life itself, but the person whose life is at stake.

While human biological life is not absolute in value from a Christian viewpoint, it is still a high value. Human life is a precious gift of God and, as such, must be treated with high regard. We are to be reverential stewards. Human life is a sacred trust because it is the necessary vehicle through which God's work is accomplished in the world. To discard or neglect human life—personal or not—that retains its potential to do God's work is to violate this sacred trust. Yet, sometimes mere life works against the person whose life it is. Sometimes it carries little potential for doing God's work because it is overwhelmed with a painful struggle to survive. In these cases, other values, including surely the love of persons, might be overriding.

It is for this reason that many Christians rightly believe that they are not obligated to stretch out their lives to the limit with all the life-saving technologies modern medicine makes available regardless of the condition of that life. God's plan for us as persons includes birth, life, and death. Physical death is not the worst thing that can happen to us. There is, as the writer of Ecclesiastes says, "a time to live, and a time to die."

For Discussion

1. A human person is more than a living organism with a particular type of genetic structure (homo sapiens). And the value of life comes from the fact that it is a gift of God to persons to be used in the service of the community of persons and God. Discuss some of the implications of this view for the issues of overpopulation and population control. Is more life always better?

2. A tough problem we face when we make decisions about whether to discontinue life-saving treatments is whether we have the right to "play God" by deciding who should be kept alive and who should not. When we make these choices, we seem to be deciding when the quality of life is worthwhile and when it is not. What are the criteria for evaluating the quality of life for another person or

for oneself? Who, if anyone, should be involved in these decisions?

3. Sometimes babies are born without brains—anencephalus—and hence have no capacity for conscious awareness. How ought we to relate to these babies? Ought we accord to them the full status of personhood and provide them with the same life-saving treatment and care we would give a baby with potential for a much higher quality of life?

3

The Clinic, the Church, and the Kingdom

Howard J. Loewen

A YOUNG CHRISTIAN couple expecting their first child learn from their physician that the woman carries a gene with a 50 percent chance of causing blindness in their male offspring. Half of the female offspring will be carriers of the defect. Through amniocentesis, physicians can tell whether the fetus likely will be blind or only a carrier of the defect. The husband and wife are trying to decide whether to have an abortion rather than risk transmitting this disorder to the children they hope to bear. If you were the pastor, parent, or physician, what counsel would you give this couple?

The Clinic

Christian communities must respond to three major trends in relation to medical ethics. The first is *decentralization*. Traditionally, medical ethics was the domain of medical professionals. However, now the conversation around the ethical issues related to medical practice includes many more people—law, government, education, the general public, the church. This is a positive development, indicating that people recognize the complexity of medical-health care and want to be more responsible for their well-being.

The second is *impersonalization*. Quality of life is a growing concern in our society. This is a result not only of the wars, revolutions, and ecological questions that have emerged, but also of the high-tech life-sustaining equipment that has accompanied medical developments. These issues have also raised interest in the quality of death. This may be seen, for example, in the hospice movement. In a sense, the developments are paradoxical. There is the high-tech side, which has brought us heart transplants, microsurgery, and artificial organs. But there also is the high-touch side, which emphasizes home care, home births, a homelike atmosphere in hospitals, low-tech birth rooms, and less surgery.

A third is the *deinstitutionalization* of medical care. Historically, society has handed over the responsibility for medical-health maintenance to the medical establishment. People have placed a significant amount of trust in medical personnel to care for them. Now, for a variety of reasons, some of that trust has eroded. There has been a corresponding shift to self-responsibility for certain areas of health care. These include concern for the environment, lifestyle, and nutrition. Some have referred to this trend as the "granola ethic," a shift of focus from sickness to wellness.

The church cannot offer simple, shortsighted solutions to the present clinical crisis. But, together with the medical community, it does have a responsibility to recognize its challenges and opportunities. The challenge for the church is to move from *quandary ethics* (deciding what to do in a crisis) to *quality-of-life ethics* (learning how to live a "shalom vision" of peace and wholeness). It has the responsibility to provide healing for both those who give and those who receive health care. Its main role is not so much to help the professional and the patient make the right decisions as to create a context of understanding, care, and support in times when tough decisions have been made or difficult realities have struck. Here are some suggestions for beginning to work at this concern:

1. As a congregation, establish links with a health care facility in your community and find ways to interact with it regularly.

2. Have a group in the congregation do a careful analysis of how many members are in a health-related profession and how many people in the past year have received major medical care because of illness or accident. Try to determine what is already going on in your congregation in regards to the interfacing of medicine and faith.

3. Encourage clergy to visit health care professionals from their congregation at their places of work so that they can get a clearer picture of the accomplishments and dilemmas of these persons. Perhaps clergy and health care providers may gain more understanding of the interconnectedness between religious tradition and modern medical practice.

4. Provide a forum for medical professionals to express the dilemmas of modern health care with which they struggle. Ask them how to say how the changes in medical technology are affecting them, and what the church can do to relate to the emerging dilemmas.

5. Help people allay their fears of medicine and hospital procedures by having persons who have faced medical crises share what happened to them. They could explain how they felt when going through the crises, and how they appreciated the skilled and caring doctors and nurses.

6. Form a congregational care group consisting of medical and nonmedical people that would work through a process by which your congregation could assist people who have difficult medical decisions to make. Show how to work through a medical dilemma by identifying the main alternatives. Assess the strengths and weaknesses of each alternative. Justify the best alternative by providing sufficient and compelling reasons for it. Finally, evaluate whether this is truly the best decision for the person(s) involved.

The Church

It is a Sunday morning in our congregation, and people are gathering for worship. I think about the congregation as a place of healing. We have those who are sick—in body, mind, and spirit—and those who care for the sick. In front of me sits a family whose young daughter recently died of leukemia after a long hospitalization and many visits and supportive gestures by friends and church members. Behind me a family enters whose teenage daughter recently survived a serious accident. She had to endure a long period of rehabilitation and needed a great deal of support from her youth group. Across the aisle a middle-aged man of robust appearance shows no signs of his brush with death after he contracted hepatitis the past year. He has a special appreciation for this congregation. A young woman in the choir has had periodic bouts with cancer and recently had a mastectomy. She continues to need much support from friends within the church. These are some of the sick who have experienced varying degrees of care from this congregation.

On the pew beside me is a nurse whose daily routine is to help people die with dignity in a hospice center. At the end of the week, he comes to the worship service to be revitalized. He represents those who care for the sick, who daily make numerous ethical decisions regarding the care of their patients and clients, and who also care about the church as a spiritual resource for their vocations. The congregation also includes several other nurses, a cardiologist, a number of mental health professionals, a pediatrician, a director of nursing-care homes, a surgeon, a gynecologist, and dental care specialists.

This is an authentic portrayal of the close relationship between health care and the church in the experience of one congregation. But it does not accurately portray what has happened to the role of the church in health care in our society. Historically, medicine received its greatest impetus from the church. Yet today most church-initiated health care endeavors are functionally indistinguishable from their secular counterparts. The church has been largely absent in health care and bioethical discussions. This neglect is beginning to be remedied. The church must be mindful of several things if it is to enhance its role in relation to health care and medicine.

Character. The church must ask what kind of community it wants to be and whether it really has anything to offer to health care issues. Mainstream religion has declined and will continue to decline in its influence on health care because of its accommodation to an increasingly secularized and technologically oriented culture. The church with a strong sense of mission for the well-being of the whole person will have a significant influence on the health care practices within its community.

Many regard illness as a private affair and guard it accordingly—often because it is an embarrassment to them. But the gift of health and the burden of disease are not private matters. The church must be involved in nurturing health care, for today's major health care issues are primarily lifestyle-related. For example, cancer, AIDS, and cardiovascular diseases involve moral issues relating to how we live. Therefore, the church must reclaim what has become an increasingly compartmentalized area of our life and once again be a shalom community ministering to the whole person.

Care. It is important to identify what the church and the clinic are actually doing to provide care for the sick and deal with difficult medical and related ethical issues. The media and the medical profession frequently focus on spectacular cases and impossible dilemmas of modern medicine. So we often do not recognize the quality of care for the sick that people are providing in a quiet inconspicuous way. Nor do we see the effective support given for the ethical decisions people need to make when sickness brings a crisis into their lives, or the spiritual care given by pastor, physician, and others. Health-related issues may provide the most opportune moments for uncovering and exploring some of the most profound spiritual and moral commitments of the church and the clinic. For example, we pray for those who are sick both in the congregation and in the clinic. There is still an unusual freedom to do that in most congregations. Such an emphasis should not be diminished.

The commitment of the clinic, and even more so the church, is to be present to the ill even when no easy answers are available to the moral and spiritual questions they ask. Yet in an increasingly pluralized and secularized society, this kind of dedication is becoming more difficult to sustain. Therefore, the burden again falls on the church as a kingdom community to call for that kind of human care and to provide people who possess that quality of caregiving.

Co-workers. The clinic and the church—specifically the pastoral care and the health care persons—must work harder to develop a partnership. The hospital and the congregation must discover how each needs the other. Such relationships have existed in the past, but now we must explore them more intentionally to ensure that cooperation continues. The church and the clinic must be co-workers in soul care for the sick. All Christians can act pastorally in bringing soul care to those who are sick and in providing an environment in which persons can make difficult decisions redemptively.

In addition, the relationship of medicine and religion is visible through the presence of medical professionals in congregations as faithful, active members along with other parishioners from all walks of life. The basic spiritual needs of medical professionals are different from those of others. They, no less than people in other callings, need a place to get their bearings as they wrestle with the failures, misjudgments, and problems peculiar to their work. The congregation is the place where the medical professional can join everyone else in laying before God the burdens that no human can bear alone.

Climate. The challenge for the church is to learn how to provide care and cure for the sick in an age of increasing economic scarcity. The crisis confronting medicine today is more financial than medical. Increasingly, the issue is a conflict between the sanctity of life and the scarcity of resources. This situation may spell a new opportunity for the clinic and the church: to care for one another in the midst of tragedy, not denying the limits of our resources or our mortality.

The aim of medicine to eliminate suffering or to prevent death must be evaluated carefully. In a technological culture the tendency is to make suffering pointless and to isolate those who are suffering. However, the church is to be a messenger of God's grace to those who suffer. For the person of religious conviction, both health and sickness have meaning. A community with a shalom vision can help persons discover this way of life and live it. In such a vision, illness is a sign that a disruption has occurred in the harmonious relationship God intended for creation and the church. Disease bears witness to the reality of sin in life, even though one should not draw a straight line from sickness to sin.

There is a veil of mystery that lies over the experience of becoming ill. The unsettling fears that accompany illness are very threatening. Yet when we are ill, we find a context and a grounding for some of life's deepest questions. This perspective is contrary to our culture's approach, which too often is the quick fix—treating the symptom, denying the inevitability of illness, and therefore fostering an unpreparedness to face it.

The church can be a significant caregiver offering another dimension. When people are ill, they need support, instruction, assurance, admonition, and the promise of God's grace. There is a special opportunity during crisis moments of pain to minister to the whole person. The church is in a unique position to point to the power of faith in a living God that does make a difference. There are even special liturgical moments (such as communion) in which one can specifically address the problems accompanying illness. This makes the congregation a unique place for bringing people who are isolated and alienated by illness back into a circle of belonging. The congregation is the setting for the practice of traditions that speak to the heart of human alienation from God and which lead people back into the fellowship with God and with one another. It is from within this understanding of health care that the church must reappropriate the apostolic injunction, "Is any one of you sick? He should call the elders of the church to pray over him and anoint him with oil in the name of the Lord" (James 5:14). This teaching finds its origins in Jesus' own ministry.

Here are suggestions to help persons within the congregation actively relate their faith to medical concerns:

1. Bring physicians, nurses, hospital administrators, and volunteers into congregational programs. Ask them to speak of what they see as the intersections of biblical faith and modern medicine. Ask them to suggest perspectives on how the church can help resolve the difficult ethical dilemmas modern medicine poses for patients and medical professionals alike.

2. Help healthy people to recognize the spiritual resources available when health gives way to illness. Help them to envision the hospital as a place where the providence of God is present.

3. Encourage people to reevaluate their attitudes toward and expectations of doctors and hospitals. Also encourage them to report serious malpractice problems without regarding litigation as the only means of such a protest.

4. Encourage laypeople to visit persons in the hospital.

5. Mobilize a small group to help the household of an ill person to continue to function through a time of acute or prolonged illness.

6. Offer assistance by donating blood, sorting through the maze of paperwork incurred in Medicare and other insurance coverage, or providing emergency financial support.

The Kingdom

When Jesus came into Peter's house, he saw Peter's mother-in-law lying in bed with a fever. He touched her hand and the fever left her, and she got up and began to wait on him.

When evening came, many who were demon-possessed were brought to him, and he drove out the spirits with a word and healed all the sick. This was to fulfill what was spoken through the prophet Isaiah, "He took up our infirmities and carried our diseases" (Matthew 8:14-17).

The most effective treatment for the present crisis in medical ethics, health care, and the church-as-caregiver must come from a kingdom perspective. This is the most basic dimension to the big picture of health care, one that is usually eclipsed in the modern medical arena. The theme of the kingdom of God is central to Jesus' ministry. It has direct reference to the healing presence and power of God and the identification of that reality with Jesus of Nazareth, the Christ. This kingdom reality both creates and alleviates crisis in the human condition.

The kingdom creates crisis to alleviate the ultimate crisis of human sin and death. As the power and presence of God in Jesus and through his Spirit, the kingdom has a disrupting effect on human life. In Jesus the kingdom erupts and effects major change. Jesus provides the power to face the question of death and to overcome it. Medically, a crisis is a change in a disease that indicates whether the result will be recovery or death. Clinically, the emphasis too frequently is on overcoming death. But in Jesus, the emphasis is the ability to face death and participate in that power that can truly overcome it. Therefore, from a kingdom perspective, a crisis can bring major, positive change.

Jesus' ministry alleviates crisis by helping us face physical and spiritual illness and death. A kingdom perspective teaches us that sickness and suffering are not valueless. The difference between a kingdom and a clinical perspective is often that the former can see suffering as a blessing of God, whereas the latter sees it as a curse, a sign of God's absence.

One of the central emphases of Jesus' kingdom ministry is the alleviation of disease, sickness, and brokenness. In Jesus, the kingdom power brings shalom—wholeness, wellness, health in face of death and tragedy. The kingdom comes where shalom thrives in the lives of the community of disciples. It is a sign of the triumph and authority over disease, the demonic, and death. The Gospels amply illustrate this by the healing stories of Jesus' ministry. There we find a clear identification with brokenness and an integration of the physical, emotional, and spiritual in Jesus' treatment of illnesses ranging from paralysis, to paranoia, to possession. The kingdom approach to crisis is holistic. It involves the spirituality of whole persons. To make people whole we must be whole people living in whole communities that are able to deal with sin, suffering, and death.

Jesus' portrayal of the kingdom in his life and ministry provides such a pattern for the church. Without this perspective, modern medicine will not be able to put the Humpty Dumpty of human brokenness back together again. The kingdom reality provides both a model and a method of treatment for our clinical and cultural crises.

The crisis of medicine today is largely spiritual and moral. Medicine has benefited us greatly; but for all its benefits, it cannot deliver us from our finiteness. The victory over disease and death, pain and tears, is a divine victory, not a technological one. Medical ethics, health care, and the Christian church must reassert an identity of care in the midst of tragedy—even when cure is not possible. We must nurture a sense of the sanctity and divine wholeness of life in the context of inevitable brokenness. The kingdom power and ethic of the church instruct us to endure and face problems holistically, not simply to solve them partially. Shalom communities must be characterized by the compassion and care that Jesus and the apostles manifested.

A central part of the legacy of Christian tradition is compassion. Followers of Jesus have shown a keen spirit of care for the needy and sick—sometimes accompanied by a certain suspicion of medicine the world practices. So they have been involved with care for the aged, the establishment of hospitals of various sorts, deaconess work, nursing education, health insurance and mutual aid, chaplaincy, wellness care, and more. Keeping alive this spiritual tradition of compassion will take us a long way in dealing with the current crises in health care and preserving the shalom vision of the kingdom. We must be a church that gives spiritual, pastoral, and moral leadership in one of the most encompassing social-ethical issues we face in our society.

Here, then, are suggestions for relating our vision of the kingdom of God to medical-health care concerns:

1. Emphasize more the centrality of healing in the church's ministry—healing of body, soul, and spirit. Establish a wellness program in your congregation to foster an emphasis on prevention. Incorporate into your communion service, or other liturgical moments, an emphasis on prayer and ministry for those who have been alienated and broken through sickness, whether in body, soul, or spirit.

2. Plan a Sunday school class on the Bible, the church, and modern medicine. Deal with modern medicine and miracles. Review the history of your tradition in relation to its contribution to health care. Review previous cases of illness in your congregation to see how you have been doing as a congregation in providing support in health care and medical-ethical decision-making.

3. Have sermons and other teaching formats that (a) encourage people to see health care as a service-oriented field of opportunity; (b) counter a view of salvation and health that merely reinforces an individualistic good life—health and wealth; (c) see the redemptive side of suffering and illness; and (d) instruct members on such practical things as living wills, durable power of attorney, and other means of preparing for death.

4. Find ways in which individuals in your congregation, or the congregation as a whole, can serve as a catalyst and a prophetic voice in your community in relation to health care issues. For example, establish a task force to evaluate the quality of care the poor receive from county hospitals.

For Discussion

1. How have you experienced the benefits and dilemmas of modern medicine?

2. In what ways have you experienced the church as a supportive and informative community in relation to medical and health care issues?

3. In what ways is your congregation building bridges between faith and medicine? What can you and your congregation do to integrate the concerns of the medical and the faith community?

4. Comment on these statements: The most significant contribution that the church can make is not to provide the right answers to all of the ethical dilemmas in modern medicine, but to support its members in sickness and in health and to assist them in making tough choices involving pain, suffering, and sadness. The church is to be a community that proclaims the wholeness of life in the midst of brokenness, that holds to the sanctity of life in the midst of tragedy.

5. How does the message of the kingdom, of eternal life, and of new life in Christ inform your dealing with the relationship between faith and medicine?

6. How have you seen the healing power of Christ and his Spirit manifested in your life and among God's people?

7. How do you view the healing ministry of Jesus? To what extent has your congregation appropriated healing as a sign of the kingdom into its life and teaching?

4

Death and Dying: Prevailing Medical Perspectives

Willard S. Krabill

MY LAST WORDS to him were at 9:30 p.m.; he died at 1:30 a.m. I wanted to kiss him, but I couldn't—his mouth held a restrictor. I wanted to hold him close, but I couldn't—there were tubes, IVs, and ties all around him. My heart was breaking, and I asked two nurses to take all of the stuff off and let him die in peace. He nodded his head in agreement. He was alert, though dying.

Where is the mercy? Where is the humanity? Where is the love? I only saw a man being forced to suffer—ready to die, yet being denied that right. The doctors just wouldn't let go.

■ ■ ■

Letting go does not come easily to physicians. Throughout their training and careers, physicians are oriented toward curing, healing, fixing. Their preparation involves little that helps them acknowledge the ultimate limitation of their profession. The story above is from a letter written by a bitter widow to her own physician, a friend of mine. It told of her painful experience at a nearby regional medical center.

Allowing to die—letting go—is one of the most dominant

issues in medical ethics. Only a minority of us will face issues related to abortion, surrogate motherhood, gene therapy, or artificial means of reproduction. Most of us, however, will face end-of-life decisions such as letting go. Our view of life, death, and dying is crucial to many of the ethical decisions we must make in relation to medical-health care.

Viewing Life

One of the reasons many of us are frustrated in dealing with the medical system is that most medical scientists and practitioners look at the human being in a fundamentally different way than does the Christian. The biomedical model is a mechanical model. The human is a machine, made up of many parts (organ systems) that can be separated out and treated by specialists. It is a biological-engineering model. The spiritual dimension, if acknowledged at all, is regarded as emotionally important but not as ultimate reality.

The Christian sees persons as spiritual, physical, emotional, and social beings, united and integrated, all dimensions interrelated and interdependent. What affects one part affects all. Medicine, on the other hand, tends to view persons in terms of cells, molecules, and organ systems—all functioning in predictable mechanical fashion. The Christian sees the person as an embodied unit whose spiritual reality is equal to and coexistent with the physical and emotional. It makes a tremendous difference in the medical decisions we make if we regard the physical as all there is. We need more than scientific knowledge to understand God's greatest creation—humankind.

One of the reasons we are faced with such tough ethical dilemmas is that research has attempted to define the human being in the laboratory without considering the ethical questions. Then we come along later and try to pick up the pieces. For example, what ethical forethought went into the decision to implant artificial hearts? What about the suggestion of some that we might "keep alive" the newly dead (neo-morts) in a special institution as sources for future organ donation, the manufacture of blood for transfusion, or as objects on which to perform surgical experiments?

Succeeding chapters in this book will deal with the meaning of life and personhood. I simply want to emphasize that how we view life and its meaning has everything to do with how we view death. It is to the medical perspective on death that we now turn.

Viewing Death

Before modern medical technology came along to blur the boundaries between being dead and being alive, the social commitment of the physician was accepted and seemed clear enough: to prolong life and relieve suffering. Now, however, even that straightforward obligation can become a dilemma. Powerful pain-relieving agents are available, but at times we cannot achieve both objectives. To gain an adequate dose of morphine—which suppresses respiration—to relieve the excruciating pain of some terminal cancer victims might shorten that person's life. Is it justifiable to shorten life to relieve suffering?

There can be some unfortunate results from medicine's preoccupation with the preservation of physical life. This potential overconcern to sustain life might really be an attempt to avoid death. We live in a society that fears death, that cannot accept death as part of life, and that makes an idol of biological—not holistic—health and existence. This view assumes that death is unnatural and that its delay through whatever medical or technical means necessary is always a positive human and scientific triumph. It assumes that prolonging life is always good.

Our failure to come to terms with death as part of life, as a society and as a profession, has led us into some grotesque practices in our modern hospitals and has resulted in the addition of very burdensome costs to our national health care expenditures. From one-fourth to one-third of all acute general hospital care is spent on persons who are dead within a year. A study of Medicare patients revealed that one-third of Medicare payments go for the care of persons who die within six months. Almost half the average cost of health care for a person's entire life may be spent during the last six months of life. The high-tech effort of keeping many critically ill people alive during that time is extremely expensive, often inappropriate, and may not even be what the individual would want.

Physicians, many believe, have a particular problem dealing with death. First, medical science seems to focus its energy on prolonging life regardless of its quality. Second, with the focus on physical life—to the exclusion of the spiritual—losing life is to lose all. When the physical is all there is, it is very hard to turn off respirators. Death is the enemy, to be avoided at all cost and by all means. Death is not a release, but the ultimate disaster.

Third, the death of a patient represents a personal professional failure, a lack of skill. Physicians tend to need to be in control; death reminds us that we are not in control. Death shows us our finiteness. Some claim that persons who have a problem accepting death tend to be attracted to the medical profession. In any case, many physicians do have a problem accepting death—their own as well as others. Last, since the technological explosion of the past forty years, physicians have become preoccupied with dramatic progress, with exciting new technology, with curing at the expense of caring. Thus, when involved with a person with a chronic or terminal illness, the physician's attention tends to lag.

This neglect of the incurably ill is one factor that has led to the growth of the hospice movement, a centuries-old concept that has been revived and has been such a blessing in the lives of thousands of dying persons and their families. Hospice care has reemphasized the importance of *caring* when *curing* is impossible. As Edwin H. Cassem, chief of the Critical Care Committee at Massachusetts General Hospital has noted, "even when we decide that our advanced technologies are no longer needed, we can still agree that certain extreme measures are indicated—extreme responsibility, extraordinary sensitivity, heroic compassion." Prolonging life is not always the best care. Caring may mean stopping painful, futile, or even unrequested treatment.

What Has Technology Done to Us?

Among the most dramatic—and the most ethically controversial—medical technological advances have been the resuscitative techniques. Premature low-birth-weight infants that formerly had no chance of surviving now are being kept alive. Both in the critically ill and the handicapped newborn, resuscitation techniques and respirators, along with new nutritional methods, enable bodies to be kept functioning indefinitely.

All of this permits us to influence greatly the time and manner of our passing, thus giving rise to a whole range of ethical dilemmas never anticipated by Hippocrates, nor by the writer of Ecclesiastes when he wrote, "There is a time to be born and a time to die" (3:2). Few diseases any longer can be said to have a natural history. And when we keep hearts beating and lungs breathing, how do we decide which degree of remaining brain function is necessary to call someone alive when he or she is in a permanent coma? Technology has so blurred the boundary between being dead and being alive that the ethical dilemma involved in deciding when to pull the plug can leave us feeling altogether helpless.

To deplore this frustration is not to suggest that all technology is bad. Medical technology, like life and death, is a gift from God—to be used in trust. We must link our capacity and zeal to create to assessing the effects of what we create. We must seriously question our worship of technology. *Can do* does not mean *should do*. The question is whether technology becomes our master or our servant. The problem lies in the power of technology to entice us into unethical actions, forgetting the temptation to misuse it and the consequences of failing to identify its inappropriate use. Technology can—and too often does—compete with compassion. It is very alluring and tends to become an end in itself.

The acceptance of technological solutions presents those who would decline their use with some real frustrations—even accusations of suicidal thoughts. If, for reasons of Christian stewardship or personal preference, I decide against the use of some life-saving procedure, should Christians consider that suicide?

When used to postpone death, we refer to technology as *life-sustaining treatment*; and the capacity has led to a call for still newer definitions of death. When I began my medical practice, the primary definition was *vital signs death*. When the heart and lungs stopped, life was over. All that I needed to determine whether death had occurred was a stethoscope and a flashlight. No more!

In the past twenty years, most states decreed that *brain death* was the criterion—the cessation of all levels of brain activity. Then along came cases like Paul Brophy and Karen Quinlan—who were not brain dead but in a permanent coma—in what is called a *chronic vegetative state*. All responses, all mental activity, everything that differentiates the human from the animal was permanently gone; however, the lowest level of the brain functioned enough to sustain the heartbeat and breathing. Their lives were maintained with artificial feeding tubes. In those cases, did the artificially (technologically) supplied food and water constitute *heroic* or *extraordinary* measures? Would stopping them be morally permissible?

There are some physicians, including some Christian physicians, who answer yes. They are calling for a new definition of death: *mind death* or *personal death*. They claim that when we permanently lose the capacity to relate to another human being, our personhood is over. Then Christian stewardship would require that we spend the million dollars that it cost to keep Karen Quinlan "alive" for ten years on the immunization of poor children, prenatal care for indigent women, and so forth. They would say Karen Quinlan actually died ten years before and that we would have done her a favor to have removed the feeding tube and allowed her to complete her dying then.

The issue becomes even more clouded when the individual is not really in coma, but yet is truly vegetative—unable to think, walk, talk, or respond in any meaningful way—for example, those aged persons for whom life has no meaning and in fact has become horribly burdensome. When such persons cannot or will not eat, is it our moral duty to force-feed them with a nasogastric tube? Is that the loving, humane thing to do? Or is that intrusive, coercive, and, in fact, forcibly taking from them their last freedom—the freedom to choose? Our response to this dilemma remains divided.

The medical profession is likewise divided. In March 1986, the Council on Ethical and Judicial Affairs of the American Medical Association (AMA) issued this statement on withholding or withdrawing medical treatment:

> The social commitment of the physician is to sustain life and relieve suffering. Where the performance of one duty conflicts with the other, the choice of the patient, or his family or legal representative if the patient is incompetent to act on his own behalf, should prevail. In the absence of the patient's choice or an authorized proxy, the physician must act in the best interest of the patient.
>
> For humane reasons, with informed consent, a physician may do what is medically necessary to alleviate severe pain or cease or omit treatment to permit a terminally ill patient whose death is imminent to die. However, he should not intentionally cause death. In deciding whether the administration of potentially life-prolonging medical

treatment is in the best interest of the patient who is incompetent to act in his own behalf, the physician should determine what the possibility is for extending life under humane and comfortable conditions and what are the prior expressed wishes of the patient and attitudes of the family who have responsibility for the custody of the patient.

Even if death is not imminent but the patient's coma is beyond doubt irreversible and there are adequate safeguards to confirm the accuracy of the diagnosis and with the concurrence of those who have responsibility for the care of the patient, it is not unethical to discontinue all means of life-prolonging medical treatment.

Life-prolonging medical treatment includes medication and artificially or technologically supplied respiration, nutrition, or hydration. In treating a terminally ill or irreversibly comatose patient, the physician should determine whether the benefits of treatment outweigh its burdens. At all times the dignity of the patient should be maintained.

This pronouncement of the AMA has been extremely controversial. A great many physicians welcomed it, mindful of the 10,000 to 15,000 permanently comatose vegetating individuals (persons?) in the U.S., as well as many thousands more forced to stay alive in nursing homes across the land. Other physicians rejected the statement because of differing ethical beliefs. Many more would not adhere to it for fear of liability lawsuits. And, in fact, such discontinuance of feeding is illegal in some states. This illustrates the quandary we are in when it comes to even this one area of letting go.

In making the decision to withdraw artificially provided food and water, an important concern is whether the individual would experience pain. Is death by starvation a painful death? From experience with dying cancer patients and in hospice situations, there is much evidence that it is not a painful death if local care and moisture are provided to lips, mouth, and eyes. The rising level of waste products in the blood seems to provide a natural sedative and pain-relieving effect. When it comes to those in deep coma, there is even greater assurance that withdrawing tube feeding does not cause pain.

Whose Right to Decide?

Over the past twenty years, there has been a growing affirmation, confirmed by numerous court decisions, that the patient has the right to determine what shall be done with and to his or her body. Karen Quinlan's parents won the right to stop her respirator—but she lived on. Paul Brophy's wife won the right to remove his feeding tube—and he died eight days later. Elizabeth Bouvia won the right to decline force-feeding—then didn't exercise her right, but sued the hospital's ethics committee!

When the patient is no longer competent or able to speak for himself, then a properly chosen surrogate may speak for him. Sometimes that surrogate is a natural or obvious choice, such as a spouse or other family member. At other times the choice may be disputed. Sometimes the courts are involved and appoint a "disinterested third party" (*guardian ad litem*) to represent the interests of the incompetent patient.

Those of us who have convictions about what we want done to or for us when we can no longer speak for ourselves should take steps to assure that our wishes are carried out. We can accomplish this through a *living will*, giving some trusted person *durable power of attorney*, or through a guardian. To do so can be an act of thoughtfulness, responsibility, and Christian stewardship.

There is an added dimension to the matter of society's emphasis on the individual's right to decide about appropriate care and high-tech treatment. The individualism of our society contradicts the life-in-community concepts precious to Christians. Knowing we are interdependent with our brothers and sisters in the family of faith, we need not make these decisions in isolation.

Conclusion

This chapter has focused on some of the ethical dilemmas surrounding our attitudes toward death and allowing to die. Modern medical technology has created serious ethical dilemmas for us. To have the power that we do to alter the time and manner of our passing is an awesome and painful responsibility, especially when we're called on to make a decision for others. The problem addressed in this chapter is the way we view life and death, living as we do in a society that both fears and denies death, viewing death as "the end" rather than as a beginning.

Death is an enemy, but it is not *the* enemy. And for Christians, it is a defeated enemy. Our never-say-die attitudes add tremendous cost to our health care bills and often add immense burden and frustration to the lives of those in their later years. In the words of an insurance company advertisement, "The fear of dying early has been replaced by the fear of living too long."

For Discussion

1. Is it justifiable—in the name of "human life is sacred and priceless"—to drain a family's or a congregation's financial resources to pay for medical care if the patient has little chance of recovering or realizing long-range benefit from prolonged treatment?

2. A physician will fear liability in withdrawing life-sustaining treatment even if the patient has a living will whenever members of the family are in disagreement. How can families arrive at one mind in making these kinds of decisions?

3. Does a hopelessly ill person, terrified of death, have the right to demand that everything be done to save his or her life if he or she is financially unable to pay for such care? What is a congregation's role in such a case?

4. If Karen Quinlan had been a member of your congregation, what would you have advised the family regarding stopping the tube-feeding?

5. If you went into an irreversible coma tonight, what would you want done to yourself? Who would you want to speak for you? Have you told that person?

6. Do you have a living will?

7. Would you want your heart donated for transplant?

8. What is life-saving medical technology? Is it not buying time rather than saving life? (No one gets out of this world alive.)

9. What, for you, is appropriate use of expensive, high-tech medical treatment? Who should receive it? Who should decide who gets what? Should age be a consideration? Should ability to pay be a consideration?

5

Life and Death: Biblical-Theological Perspectives

David Schroeder

GOD IS the author of life because God is life. That is, God "has life in himself" (John 5:26) and bestows life on others. God is the *living* God and is known as such in the Bible (Deuteronomy 5:26; Matthew 26:63; Romans 9:26; Revelation 7:2). We understand what the Bible calls *life* only in terms of the God who lives and bestows life on others (1 Samuel 14:39).

The Creation of Life

Humans are related to the created order. The creation accounts—Genesis 1:1-2:4a and 2:4b—3:24)—highlight three things about human creatureliness. (1) Humans were formed out of the dust of the earth, as were trees and other animals (2:9, 19). (2) Humans, animals, fish, and birds received the "breath of life" (1:30; 2:7, 19). (3) Physical life terminates in physical death and ends when the breath of life is taken away (Psalm 104:29).

Humans also are related to God; they are created "in the image of God" (Genesis 1:26-27). Humans stand in a special relation to God; they are God's representatives on earth. This representation finds its fullest expression in Jesus, the Son of God incarnate (Colossians 1:15; 2 Corinthians 4:6). To be representatives of God on earth implies a quality of life that is more than biological or physical life. For God's representatives to have life means for them to be truly and fully human.

The first and most obvious mark of true humanity is accepting and fulfilling the tasks God assigned to God's representatives on earth: to be co-creators with God in the birthing of children and to have dominion over the created order (Genesis 1:28). Humans are to assist God in governing and giving shape to the world.

A fully human life involves our being persons who, as moral agents, are responsible in relation to God, others, and the world about us; who are free to make choices; and who take responsibility for our actions. As moral, free, and responsible beings, we are called to engage in meaningful, purposeful work that is in harmony with the purposes of God in creation.

As Adam was called upon to name the animals, so all humans are engaged in naming the world. Through various disciplines of study, we analyze and classify and name things so that we can order the world for ourselves and others. Our actions call into being a material world (what we build and destroy), a cultural world (what we value in life), and a spiritual world (what we believe, our worldview). To have fully human life, these aspects of naming and ordering life must be in the direction of God's will and end.

To have truly human life involves community. The family is the basis for a much larger community of relationships. The creation account stresses that humans were not meant to be alone, but to live in community with each other (Genesis 2:18). To have life is to be related to others under God.

Finally, as implied in all of the above, to have truly human life is to be rightly related to the Creator. God created the world with a purpose. God evaluated the creation as good (Genesis 1:4, 21, 31). Only life that is lived in harmony with the will of God is true life and thus good. God set the moral direction of the world. It is up to God's human representatives on earth to discern this direction and to act on it. To do so is to choose life.

Life is much more than mere biological life. Life refers to a quality of living, a way of being that is in harmony with God's purpose in creation.

The Entrance of Death

Humans were free moral agents. The more humans exercised their God-given responsibilities of dominion, the more they desired to know good and evil. The more they knew good and evil, the more they were tempted to become like God, having sovereign rule. The more they acted in their own understanding, the more they were inclined to forget that they were to be managers of the world *under God*.

The creation narrative of Genesis 3 uniquely portrays this dilemma. The serpent, part of the created order over which humans were to exercise dominion, tempted them with respect to their human limits. They were not to eat of the fruit of the tree of the knowledge of good and evil. With the eating of the fruit, they became like God. That is, they now knew good and evil. They were not gods; but on the basis of the knowledge of good and evil, they could now act according to their own notions of right and wrong. As a consequence, they felt they no longer needed God. By separating themselves from God, they brought death—the opposite of true life—into the world.

The focus here is not so much on biological death—they did not immediately die a physical death—but on death entering the sphere of life. The idyllic situation was seen in terms of biological life and biological death both being in the direction of true life. Now, because of sin, biological life and biological death moved in the direction of death and threatened to overcome true life. Now life was in need of God's redemption.

Sin changed things. Sin separated all things from their intended purposes. It separated them from the true life God gave and made them instruments of death. Death as separation from God entered the lives of the living because of sin and disobedience. Death entered because humans no longer respected the will and purposes of God.

What happened when death entered the lives of the living? What really changed?

The first change was that biological life and biological death were no longer directed toward the quality of life God intended for humankind. Because humans made choices that ran counter to

God's purposes, they moved in directions that were contradictory to God's purposes of life, what God had defined as good. Because their living was no longer oriented toward life, people began to fear biological death. The result of sin was that humans could no longer clearly discern true life in the midst of living because death had entered their lives. Nor could they distinguish between physical death and death as separation from God.

With the entrance of sin, human dominion changed. Humans now governed and managed in accordance with their own purposes and designs. They could now do without God. As a consequence, their actions led to conflict, subjugation, destruction, and death (Genesis 3:16b; 4:8, 23-24; chaps. 6-9, 11), not life. Humans are still working to till and keep the garden, but it has turned into an eco-logical nightmare, threatening life on earth. Humans are still in the process of naming the world, but so much of it is not truthful. Our advertising is naming as good and desirable a world of materialism, luxury, wealth, and power; but it is a lie. To name the most deadly bombs *peacemakers* is to put the wrong name on death. So little of the naming of the world is truthful and in the direction of life. The shades of death are everywhere.

Humans are still co-creators with God in the birthing of children; but here too problems of death have entered life. Questions of birth control, birthing practice, abortion, genetic screening, and organ transplants need careful deliberation and evaluation. What constitutes decision and action in the direction of life is not always easy to determine.

Humans are still co-creators with God in shaping a material and cultural world. The world that will be in the future will be determined by our choices and actions today. By many seeking to become rich, others have been impoverished. By some seeking control through power and might, others have been enslaved. By threatening each other with death, the whole world is on the threshold of death. Sin does not lead to life, but to death.

Humans still live in community, but the human community is disrupted by sin. Wife-husband relationships are in jeopardy. Parent-child relationships are deteriorating. Society, seeking protection from criminal actions, calls for the death penalty. The moral fiber of nations erodes through a pluralism of religions and worldviews, so that effective and just lawmaking is impossible. Individualism is encouraged through more calls for freedom, and any counter moves are branded as communistic. Unjust standards of living are enforced by national policies of power and military might. Everywhere we find the shades of death!

Death has entered all spheres of life because there is no longer the proper worship and praise of God. There is no longer a regard for the order God created and the good ends and purposes God had in mind. Through human disregard for the life God gave, sin and death have entered the land of the living.

God Creates New Life

The acts of God. From the beginning, God is the Author of life and continues to work toward true life in the midst of a sinful world. God does not seek the death of the sinners, but rather seeks to give them life.

The actions of God toward life are well known. God clothes the rebellious humans and protects them from eating the tree of life (Genesis 3:21-24). God protects Cain from his enemies (4:15) and Noah from destruction (6:11—8:22). God gives new life through his promises of life to those who follow his bidding (12:1ff.). God frees the slaves of an oppressive Pharaoh (Exodus 3:1ff.) and makes a covenant with them, binding them to God's will.

The laws that God gave to the people were a reflection of the character of God and a manifestation of the life God offers to all humankind. These laws came to the defense of the poor, the slave, the stranger, the widow, and the orphan. All those who were helpless and powerless to defend themselves were given God's protection and help. The law revealed a loving God who at all times sought the good of his people in giving them the possibility of true life.

In the two actions of God—the freeing from bondage and the call to keep the commandments of God—we have a description of the ongoing loosing and binding activity of God. God frees people from bondage to sin and to the principalities and powers of evil, so that they may bind themselves to what will bring life.

The work of God through the prophets represents another way in which God continually works toward life. God gave the prophets insight into the life of the people. They saw that under the guise of religion, people did all kinds of things that were not in harmony with the covenant God had made with them and were producing death, not life. Their word and their call for repentance caused people to turn again to God and live.

Life in Christ. The manifestation of the fullness of life came in Jesus Christ, the Son of God incarnate, recognized by early Christians as the new Adam (Romans 5:12-21; 1 Corinthians 15:22, 45; Philippians 2:5-11). He revealed his dependence on and obedience to God and was tempted and tested as are other humans (Matthew 4:1ff.; Hebrews 4:14ff.; 5:2ff.). He lived in the real world and shared fully in our human experiences, including physical death. He took on the form of a servant, not a despot (Mark 10:42-45). Since he lived in perfect obedience to God—his sinlessness is noted repeatedly (2 Corinthians 5:21; 1 Peter 2:22)—he is the manifestation of what truly human life is.

Jesus also was the true representative of God. As Paul says, "he is the image of the invisible God, . . . for God was pleased to have all his fullness dwell in him" (Colossians 1:15, 19). Jesus fulfilled perfectly the commission given to humankind at creation: he fulfilled the will of God; he sought first the kingdom of God; he manifested the character of God in his love, justice, and forgiveness.

Jesus chose life—true life—and shared that life with others. He gave himself for others so that they too might have life (Mark 10:45). He freed people from the bondage of sickness (1:32-34), possession (5:1ff.), rejection (1:40ff.; 2:15-17), and called them to become his disciples (8:34ff.). In giving women the opportunity to sit at the feet of a teacher (Luke 10:38-42) and to commit themselves to the will of God, he accepted women as morally mature and responsible persons. Jesus is the way, the truth, and the life; and he came so that people might have life (John 14:6).

Jesus' living was death-defeating. He challenged evil with good. He loved and forgave those who persecuted him. He challenged falsehood with the truth of God and asked people to accept the truth and live. He challenged hypocrisy by exposing it and offered in its place a life of honesty, integrity, and devotion to God. He challenged the legalistic interpretation of the Scriptures and helped people to discern the truth of God as revealed in Scripture.

He challenged the structures of the law as taught by the scribes of the Pharisees and gave hope to those who despaired of ever being able to keep the law as interpreted. He challenged the wall of partition that had been built up between the Jews and the non-Jews—the Samaritans and the Gentiles (Luke 10:29ff.; John 4). Jesus broke with the patriarchal structure of the family and society and called on those who would be great in the kingdom to become the servant of all (Mark 10:39-45). He himself washed the disciples' feet (John 13:1ff.).

Above all, Jesus challenged death by accepting suffering and death rather than disobeying God. This is the most surprising challenge to the rule of death. When he was persecuted in the name of religion, he accepted it. First Peter 2:22-23 describes it vividly: " 'He committed no sin, and no deceit was found in his mouth.' When they hurled their insults at him, he did not retaliate; when he suffered, he made no threats. Instead, he entrusted himself to him who judges justly."

Jesus' actions were deliberate. He did not pay back evil for evil. He accepted suffering and physical death and in so doing unmasked the power of death. It had no hold on his life. No earthly power can do more than cause physical death. The martyr knows that the powers of death are helpless against the power of an obedient life. Though Jesus faced physical death, he knew that God would vindicate the death of the righteous and entrusted himself to God.

New symbols of life. A whole range of new symbols for life are given in the revelation of Jesus Christ.

1. New birth. Jesus indicated that new life comes by being born of the Spirit (John 3:5), for it is the Spirit who gives life (6:63). Even the most pious and devout of the scribes of the Pharisees, such as Nicodemus, needed to be born again. A new turning to Christ in faith, trust, and obedience was necessary to receive newness of life. The new birth is the entrance to life.

2. Discipleship. Those who have received the Spirit are called upon to follow Jesus, to accept him as Lord in their lives. This involves carefully discerning the will of God through the reading of Scriptures, prayer, and mutual encouragements and admonition. Disciples are learners. They take Christ as their example and manifest his spirit and love in their living (John 14:12, 23-24). Jesus

frees those who follow him from captivity to death and gives them life.

3. Suffering servant. The one who is born again, who has received the Spirit of Christ, and who manifests the Spirit of Christ, will live a self-sacrificial life, just as Jesus did. Such a person will know that the model for life is the suffering servant. The servant will accept wrong without retaliation, violence, or hatred, and will forgive the wrong inflicted by others. The servant of God will absorb violence rather than amplify or multiply it. The servant will be subject to others in the name of Christ. To suffer with Christ is to have life.

4. The cross. As a new symbol, the cross stands for accepting death and the violence of death rather than to become unfaithful to God (Matthew 5:11-12; 1 Peter 2:22-23; Acts 5:29). It represents the courage of obedience to God in the midst of opposition and the threat of physical death. It symbolizes that the powers of darkness cannot prevail against the person who is in Christ and receives life from him. Jesus himself declared life that comes through death (John 12:24).

5. Resurrection. When physical death becomes the door to a new and eternal life, death has been overcome. Peter states that we have been born anew to "a living hope through the resurrection of Jesus Christ from the dead" (1 Peter 1:3). The resurrection is the sign of Christ's victory over death. We have now the assurance that since he lives, we too shall live. Death has been overcome, and there is the prospect of life for all who will receive Christ as Savior and Lord (1 Corinthians 15:20ff.).

The resurrection is the power for new life. The hope in life here and now, and in the hereafter, gives Christians the power and the strength to live by the truth of the gospel in the face of death.

For Discussion

The following comments and questions may help you discover some of the implications of biblical views of life and death for how we respond to medical crises that demand that we make difficult choices. Others may emerge as you read and discuss other chapters of this book.

1. Humans have been given the task of managing and shaping

the created order. One area in which we exercise this dominion is medicine. We can be thankful for the work that has been and is being done in this area. But all such action should be in the direction of life. Even the help we give the dying should be in the direction of true and full human life, not just physical life.

We ought to distinguish more clearly between physical life and death and the life God seeks for all persons. Physical death is really not the enemy of life, only the end of biological life. Life is not ultimately affected by physical death because physical death cannot separate us from God (Romans 8:38).

Recall a medical crisis that you might have been involved with. Was the goal to enhance life in its fullest and most truly human sense, or primarily to prolong only physical life? How might our sickness care system operate differently if we saw death not just as physical death but as the opposite of all that is most truly human? How might the medical crisis that you remembered have been different?

2. Discerning what belongs to life and what belongs to death is necessary, but not always easy. Let me illustrate. With respect to abortion, we now have two opposing camps: pro-choice and pro-life. If we view the issue from a Christian point of view, however, we have to be pro-choice (because God has created us as free moral and responsible agents) *and* pro-life (because God has called us to choose life). What belongs to life in a given situation is not always self-evident.

How would you bring together these two sides if counseling a teenager with an unwanted pregnancy? How would you do it if counseling a couple who planned the pregnancy but learned through genetic screening that the child likely will have a very brief and painful life and now are considering abortion?

3. It is extremely difficult to make ethical decisions about life and death in a pluralistic society. Is it really possible for the medical profession to take other than an individualistic base for ethics? What is needed is Christian communities where corporate discerning takes place—communities in which we free each other from methods, techniques, and actions that belong to death and bind each other to those actions that belong to life.

Are the structures for discernment within your congregation

adequately developed? If not, what steps might the congregation take to improve them before a major crisis occurs?

4. In our medical practice, we are creating a material, cultural, and spiritual world—a care system. Are we creating a system that we want to live with, or that is life-giving? We are spending an inordinate amount of money and effort in a sickness care system. How might we put more emphasis on preventing actions that we know to be direct causes of sickness and death—smoking, alcohol, drugs, AIDS-related activities, lifestyle issues? Are there political and legal channels that we should pursue, in addition to moral persuasion?

5. We ought to name much more carefully what belongs to death and what belongs to life in relation to:

a. Procreation (e.g., birth control methods, abortion, in vitro fertilization, embryo research, control of DNA, and sterilization);

b. Prolonging life and the process of dying (e.g., extraordinary means of sustaining life, resuscitation, use of drugs, and maintaining intensive-care units); and

c. Personal choice on the part of the patient (e.g., use of living wills, durable power of attorney, organ donation, and choice in treatment options and the extent of treatment).

As you proceed through this book, continue to ask, How do I discern what belongs to life and what belongs to death?

6. The church should give leadership in naming and overcoming the principalities and powers of darkness operating in our modern society. Try to name the most prominent structures of death in our society: materialism, individualism, search for security and excessive comfort, fear of death, placing more and more stock in science and technology and less stock in the personal and spiritual aspects of human life. How might Christians, individually and collectively, counter these in relation to medical-health care?

6

Maneuvering in the Health Care System

Tana Durnbaugh

RECENTLY IN OUR community, early one morning the attendants at a local gas station found the popular young owner of the station on the floor of the garage. Immediately they called the local rescue squad. The paramedics used all the latest mobile technology to maintain vital functions while transporting him to the hospital. The specialist in emergency techniques and the emergency room staff promptly initiated supportive care. They consulted with neurologic specialists. Within several hours, they began sophisticated medical interventions and monitoring techniques. Soon they decided that complex and elaborate brain surgery was necessary. Intensive-care equipment and professional procedures surrounded the patient and the family. Decisions were being made on an hourly basis—crucial decisions about how much treatment, when, and where.

The family had normal health with little extended relationships with the health care system. The community, while supportive, was not prepared to spend days at the bedside providing counsel. After surgery, the young man never regained consciousness but continued to have heartbeat and respiration. He was transferred to a long-term care agency in our town. Several months later, when the

family was exhausted emotionally and financially, the wife peti-
tioned the courts to stop the daily feedings that kept her husband
alive. She stated that this would have been her husband's wish. She
did not indicate how she knew this to be true. After extensive court
proceedings, the feedings were stopped. He died about two weeks
later.

Lack of knowledge of how the health care system works leaves
people inadequately prepared to manage the demands of negotiat-
ing the system at the point of medical crisis. In this chapter, I
consider factors that impact decision-making in the health care
system.

Obstacles to Patients Influencing
Health Care Decisions

Within the health care system, how persons define and in-
terpret health influence how they make health care decisions. Is
health a right or a privilege? While we may debate the answer to this
question, the reality is that health is a basic human need. Grand-
mothers are quick to say, "Be happy; you have your health." Insurance companies attempt to place a financial value on loss of a
limb or eye. Consider for a moment the value you place on health.
Ask yourself these questions:

1. Do I make a planned effort to care for my body?
2. How do I feel when someone I know is sick?
3. How would I feel about being sick for extended periods?

The value individuals place on health varies. Some people are
self-caring and place a high value on health promotion. Others are
less self-caring, as can be seen in such stress-related health problems
as hypertension, obesity, and drug abuse. Health values are central
to health choices and to health ethics.

We all have values, and these values influence our ethical decision-making. As Christians, our faith perspectives impact our
health values. Our values determine how we handle complex health
care dilemmas. These values help us identify acceptable alternatives
for each dilemma. These values also direct us to action based on
what we hold as essential for meaningful life.

In difficult ethical matters, we must attempt to understand the
feelings and values of all concerned, be accountable for our own

beliefs, and understand that others have the right of individual freedom. Health care decisions made at the point of crisis are complex choices based on fundamental values. As such these decisions are some of the most difficult ones we make.

Our values relative to health care may conflict with other values we hold or with those of others. Consider the World Health Organization's definition of health: "a state of complete physical, mental, and social well-being." If we define health in this manner, then we imply that health is part of social concerns like unemployment. Is this truly an area of health?

Promoting well-being is a primary concern of health care, but it is unclear to what degree. If we imply that certain behaviors, such as exercise, are healthy, do we then consider people who do not exercise regularly unhealthy? If we view smoking as unhealthy, do we consider nonsmokers as healthier and therefore better? Health is value-laden for both the patient and the health care worker.

While the patient should be the center of the decision-making process, in reality, other influences affect decision making. Some people value health for all people at any cost. Yet it is clear that all patients are not treated the same. One of the major reasons for this is the rising cost of health care—now 10 percent of the gross national product of the United States. Health care costs have increased because more people have access to health care than prior to the 1960s. New technologies have spread more quickly and more widely than in the past, and the people generally are living longer.

By treating the sick in the most cost-effective manner, some people do not receive the same care as others. The most graphic example is Medicare's regulation of the length of hospital stays by type of illness. If you have Medicare, the type of condition you have restricts the number of paid hospital days available to you. However, if you have private insurance, no such restriction applies to your hospital stay. These and other policy regulations of government or specific hospitals restrict the amount a patient can participate in health care decisions.

Patients often find themselves in high-technology settings where medical jargon is the basis of conversation. They may have little knowledge of their illness and the methods of treatment. This lack of knowledge leaves them vulnerable and unable to monitor or participate fully in the care they receive.

The primary fact that patients are ill reduces their ability to participate in decision-making. Think about your attitudes, feelings, and behavior when you are sick. Ask yourself these questions:

1. When I am sick, do I think about weighty issues of life and death?

2. When a loved one is ill, do I have the energy to talk to twelve or more people a day?

People who are ill take on a sick role. In our society, we excuse them from normal responsibilities and duties. They are allowed to be less involved. We expect them to acknowledge and to tell others that they are sick. And it is appropriate that sick people are somewhat dependent and have some level of self-concern. The energies of the sick person need to be focused toward self and self-care. However, this sick role makes a patient less able to participate in value-laden discussions of health choices.

In the past, the health professional frequently made these choices for the patient as part of his or her professional duty. While this situation was true for all health professionals, the most glaring example was in the patient-physician relationship. Historically, physicians have held a unique authority role in our society. They were expected to maintain a certain level of moral character, to possess a knowledge of medicine and healing, and to exhibit a sense of authority—a kind of charisma. We trusted dcoctors to do the best for the patient.

However, the very factors that make physicians useful also may make them dangerous. Many physicians are firmly committed to medicine as a life and accept an almost priestly devotion to it. Given this attitude, these doctors think that they are in the best position to make decisions. The paternalistic pattern of thinking and acting that may result often leads to withholding or modifying information that should be shared with the patient or the patient's family. The rationale they offer is that it is for the patient's good.

Alice was a middle-aged woman with a history of psychiatric problems, little education, and no family support. After initial tests, the doctor determined that Alice should have surgery with possible breast removal. During evening rounds, the nurse talked with Alice about her surgery the next day. Alice indicated the doctor told her not to worry—that it was only an initial procedure. The nurse confronted the surgeon, who indicated that he felt Alice could not decide what to do and that the surgery needed to be done. Consider the following:

1. Can disclosure of information be harmful to a patient?

2. Does a health care worker have the right to behave paternalistically toward patients?

3. Do you know people who act in a paternalistic manner? Can you justify their behavior?

Discussions of the relationship between the patient and the health care giver often center on issues of full disclosure of information and truth telling. Because health professionals are committed to the patient's well-being and wish to avoid inflicting harm, they may avoid the total truth. The effect of the Civil Rights era of the 1960s on health care has been the demand for equal and participatory patient roles. This is a factor in increasing malpractice suits and open debate of privacy issues related to who has access to medical records and patient information.

The ability of the patient to make decisions is based on autonomy (that is, being able to determine a course of action) and on access to adequate information. Given these two factors, a patient can make a decision. However, to carry out that decision, the attitude within the health care system must be to support the patient's decision-making. Health professionals do not need to agree with every decision, but they must be willing to participate in the decision the patient has made. In decisions related to health values, this is very difficult. Because health care providers are seldom trained in identifying or assisting patients in making ethical decisions, rarely does this permissive atmosphere exist.

Doctors recently diagnosed Sam, age seventy-six, as having cancer. His physician recommended that Sam receive a medication. After reading about the drugs and talking to others, Sam decided to refuse the treatment. The nurse, whom Sam knows and likes, believes the treatment could be successful.

1. Should health professionals always ask the patient to consent to treatment?

2. In a case like this, what are the duties of the nurse toward the patient?

In summary, a variety of factors impinge on the patient's ability to participate in decision-making. However, as pressures mount from various groups, health care providers are beginning to realize that ethical decisions must be addressed by a broader community than simply persons within the health care system.

Knowing about Health and Managing Choices in Health Care

1. *Know yourself.* The first step in managing health care choices is to decrease the number of choices that you might need to make. Healthful living and stress reduction decrease the need for medical care. If you are healthy, the problems you will eventually encounter will be similar to those of your mother and father. Consider what diseases and health problems they developed, and design a life pattern to resist these problems. Did your father have heart disease? Consult a heart specialist for advice. Become a self-caring person and take control of your health while you are healthy.

2. *Know your health resources.* The primary health resource for most people is their physician. Select your physician wisely. One woman complained about her doctor because he rushed and did not answer her questions. When asked why she continued to go to him, she answered that he was close to home. However, when she became seriously ill, the physician's habits did not change, and she had no energy to "shop around" for someone else.

Based on your health history, be a smart consumer. If you have a history of heart disease, select a physician with special skills in treating that problem. No health professional is an expert in all areas of medicine. Ask your physician to give you information about drugs, treatment alternatives, second opinions, and the use of consultants.

Health professionals have personal and professional guidelines of conduct based on professional codes of ethics. These ethical codes reflect the values of the health professional group. Beyond the code is a sense of personal commitment to the patient. Relationship at this level leads to a sense of loyalty and mutual trust, or a covenant. It is the duty of both the health professional and the patient to work toward this level of understanding and relationship. Only then can health care be truly participatory.

3. *Know your legal rights in the health care system.* Legal issues deal with malpractice, incompetence, and negligence. The law is concerned with conduct and the good of the community as a unit. Ethics deals with individual good, which may or may not apply to the larger community. Ethics involves matters of conscience and is concerned with motive and attitudes.

Licensed health professionals are bound by state regulatory bodies to adhere to certain practices. They must not take addicting drugs and must identify known child abuse. They are to adhere to these legal mandates for safe practice.

Talk to people with multiple health care experiences with different doctors and health care agencies. Various health professionals are concerned about patient's rights. "The Patient's Bill of Rights" is one group's attempt to increase patients' awareness of their rights in the health care system. Ask health care agency administrators to talk to groups you know about their agency policies to maintain patients' rights.

Knowing your legal rights will go a long way toward protecting your rights in decision-making. You should question situations that appear unusual to you and make sure that you understand your treatment, its effects, and any forms you sign related to health care. Have a lawyer talk to you or a group you work with about health care and the law.

Preparing for Health Care Dilemmas

When it comes to health care decisions, caregivers should honor the wishes of the patient. Health professionals should take the initiative in discussing with patients their desires, but it is the patient's responsibility to inform others of their decisions. The wise patient or health professional seeks the counsel of others when faced with an ethical dilemma.

One way that an individual can legally attempt to assure decision-making power is through the use of advance directives, most specifically the *living will*. These documents allow individuals to state a preference for *no heroic measures*. Despite their popularity, their legal force is uncertain. First, it is uncertain if health professionals must carry out the terms of the living will. To counter this concern, some states have enacted *natural death acts*. However, the only patients who are truly covered by this act are those who are on the edge of death despite medical intervention. People who will have a prolonged death are not affected. Of the states with natural death acts, only Delaware provides for an assigned agent for medical decision-making if the patient becomes incompetent. *Durable power of attorney* offers a powerful device for patients to continue their wishes.

Advance directives can serve as an educational device to stimulate discussion about life-saving treatments. However, before they can be used widely, several issues need resolution. First, some method must be designed to assure the competence of persons when they sign such documents. Second, the documents must assure that health professionals following their directives are not later subject to criminal liability. Third, the person who will act as the patient's proxy must be selected by some as-yet-undefined standard. Last, certain questions of administration need to be addressed: What are the time restraints on these documents? How may they be initiated? How are decisions arrived at when some third party contests the document? These and other issues need to be considered in the use of advance directives. Consider having a lawyer and a physician discuss the use of advance directives in your area.

A second, and perhaps the most effective, way to assure that patient choice is supported is advocacy. The advocate pleads the cause of the patient. Given the various barriers to patient decision-making, the advocate supports the client's decision and calls for its hearing in the health care system. Various groups have identified themselves as patient advocates.

Self-help groups intend to meet special needs or purposes. Frequently problem-oriented groups (like OWL—Older Women's League) or disease-oriented groups (like Make Today Count—cancer support groups) have ethical concerns that bring people together. Part of what they provide is advocacy for their particular ethical concerns.

Friends can be advocates. By way of a mutual agreement, friends can advocate for each other. However, it is important to realize that in the most difficult ethical dilemmas, the advocate-friend will be under tremendous stress.

Several professional health groups consider advocacy as part of their professional role. Specifically, social work and nursing identify patient advocacy as their concern. However, the conflict between the roles of patient advocate and health team member has not been resolved by these groups.

Acknowledging the complexities of ethical questions related to medical-health care, some hospitals have established ethics committees, as recommended by the American Hospital Association. The purpose of such committees is to educate and consult with health professionals on difficult decisions of patient care. Find out if your local hospital has an ethics committee. Talk to someone who is on the committee about its purpose and function.

For the patient's choice to be best served, advocates must recognize the person within the patient. They must keep uppermost the inherent dignity of the individual. They must also see that person within a context of caring. Advocates must care for and about the person. They must asknowledge their interrelatedness to the person and understand their own and the person's moral values. It would appear that the local congregation is in a unique situation to provide advocacy for ethical dilemmas.

Mennonite Brethren pastor Nick Rempel suggests that for the faith community to provide support during medical crises, it needs to be identified as a loving, supportive community of faith prior to a crisis. Then the congregation needs to support the individual or family by frequent visits, listening time, and loving prayer intervention by both the pastor and lay persons. The congregation may discuss decision-making options, but the final responsibility must stay with the individual. Members of the congregation may advocate for the individual by asking questions or contacting various health professionals. After the individual or family has made its decision, the congregation continues prayer support, frequent visits, and statements of encouragement.

Rempel indicates that the real dilemma may occur after the decision as individuals question whether they have made the correct decision. This example of congregational rapport, relationship, responsibility, and reinforcement is worthy of further discussion by churches. The church needs to assist people to explore openly the ethical conflicts of health care and support them with a caring response.

For the health care community, the patients, and their families, ethical questions require adequate knowledge of medicine and ethical decision-making processes. Unfortunately, this combination is seldom present at the time of crisis. The church can respond to this need in creative and determined advocacy for persons facing medical-health crises. What greater challenge for the caring community of faith?

For Discussion

1. If you have not done so, think about and discuss the questions that appear at various points in the chapter.

2. Find out what provisions your state government has made for living wills or durable power of attorney for health care. Try to get copies of actual legal documents and discuss them with an attorney.

7

Prolonging Life, Prolonging Death

Jesse H. Ziegler

JOHN AND LEAH have two children, ages four and seven. They live on a farm 150 miles from a large city with a children's medical center. When Leah gives birth to their third child, they are aware that something is seriously wrong even before their doctor tells them. The child's spinal cord is not completely enclosed and the brain case is still partly open. The doctor tells them that without immediate surgery in a well-equipped center for children, the baby will probably die within months or certainly a year, perhaps even days. There is no certainty of the quality of life that will result even with surgery. He asks if they want to try to save the baby.

Steve and Eleanor, both in their late seventies, have been married for fifteen years. Both have children by prior marriages. Steve is relatively frail, and Eleanor has been developing Alzheimer's disease over several years. Last year when Steve could no longer care for Eleanor in their home, he placed her in a nursing home. Eleanor has become increasingly angry and hostile toward Steve and everyone. She says she would like to die. Prior to the first indications of the disorder, both Steve and Eleanor had prepared living wills. Now Eleanor does not want to eat, but Eleanor's children want to do everything possible to keep her alive. Steve thinks it would be more in keeping with Eleanor's expressed desire to give her good care but to let non-eating take its course.

■ ■ ■

We face totally different questions in relation to medical care than did our parents and grandparents. For the most part this change has come about because of changes in technology that now make it possible to prolong life significantly and, thereby, the process of dying. Increased life expectancy is a result, but the quality and meaning of that life have not always kept pace with the additional years. The most pressing questions relate to life-threatening accidents or terminal illnesses and problems associated with newborns.

Terminal illnesses raise the question of whether we should use every means possible to keep a person alive—even when the physician believes there is no cure for the patient. When is it appropriate to forgo additional therapy? Stopping medical treatment does not mean failing to provide tender loving comfort and care for the dying person. The decision not to prolong dying means not to encumber the dying process with tubes, machines, and toxic chemicals. The choice of how to die is not dissimilar to many other choices—nature of diet, kind of exercise, place for vacation, kinds of friends.

Some persons include the choice of death itself. Hence they believe that for various reasons a person may actively seek death. They argue that there is no substantial moral difference between making available a toxic death-inducing agent to a dying person faced with intolerable pain and removing life-sustaining machines. Others believe that there is a significant ethical difference and that it feels very different to the family member who is providing care. It must be clear that the law prohibits providing death-inducing agents.

Some believe that the difference between choosing life and acquiescing in dying is theological. They hold that life is a gift of God and that we are not to throw it back in the face of the Giver. This may mean accepting the more difficult corollary that God sends—or permits—death.

An accident that results in the prospect of intolerable pain or disfigurement, loss of higher functions due to irreparable damage to the central nervous system, or loss of physical and mental functions so as to make independent life impossible raises the same questions as those facing persons with terminal illnesses. Do we let nature take its course without medical treatment, providing only for the comfort of the victim, recognizing that the individual might need such care for decades? Should we help the person to die quickly? Should the suffering person actively seek death?

Most babies are born well formed, and no question arises about providing medical care. But there are exceptions. For example, the birth of a baby with Down's syndrome—an uncorrectable condition—may raise serious questions about prolonging life because many Down's syndrome babies have other defects that are correctable surgically. This was the case of the Baby Doe in Bloomington, Indiana, which became a national incident when the parents and the primary doctor decided not to perform the surgery that would have saved the baby's life.

Cases of spina bifida—an incomplete enclosing of the spinal column during the development of the fetus—raise in a much more serious manner the question of whether to maintain the life of the child. In severe cases, the chances for life beyond six or eight months are small. But a rare case exists where, with aggressive treatment, the person lived to assist in medical research. Should we view such severely affected babies as having been born dying and therefore not treat them? Or should we treat them as if their prospective life is three weeks, three months, six months? If the baby is going to die in a few days, should there be treatment? If the wound is such as to promise repeated surgical procedures in a prospective lifespan of six months, should we provide treatment?

Who Makes Life-and-Death Decisions?

In modern relations between patients and medical caregivers, the competent patient is responsible for deciding whether to accept treatment to prolong life or dying. Certainly the patient makes such decisions in consultation with the physician on the basis of the best information provided. But the patient may also refuse the advice of the physician. The competent patient has that right. Some ethicists hold that the right should include the option of choosing an active or even an assisted approach to death in cases of intolerable pain or no possibility of improvement. Others view this as suicide or homicide.

The incompetent patient cannot make a decision because of illness or defect. Normally the family, in consultation with the physician, decides whether to treat or to let this person die. The decision may be easier if the patient has prepared a *living will* prior to becoming incompetent. In the absence of such a document, the persons who must decide should draw on what the patient may have expressed and on what they believe the person would now desire if able to express such desires. Some prefer to create a *durable power of attorney*, which legally delegates decision-making power to a person they trust to act in their best interest should they become incompetent.

But who makes decisions for the newborn? In the past physicians made such decisions—and continue to do so, though with greater consultation with the parents. But since Baby Doe and similar cases, the decision not to save the baby sometimes has been taken out of the hands of physicians and parents and claimed by the government under the necessity of protecting the rights of those unable to protect themselves. Thus courts and administrative agencies have essentially become part of the decision-making process regarding what shall happen to defective babies.

What Are the Ethical Principles for Decisions?

In his book *A Theory of Medical Ethics* (Basic Books, 1981), Robert M. Veatch provides a balanced statement of ethical principles applicable to medical questions. Most statements of ethical principles are similar, some leaning more heavily toward one principle than others.

1. *Do good.* The basic moral law governing human relationships is the obligation to do good for others—the principle of beneficence. To the extent that the principle is applied only to the person immediately at hand—for example, in the relationship of the physician and the patient—the principle may seem much too individualistic. A more thorough understanding of the principle must include a consideration of the benefit to others as well and achieve

some kind of balance among the various interests.

2. *The patient has a right to choose.* From a theological view and from the viewpoint of a rational social contract, it is the individual patient who has a right to make decisions about treatment. Consent to treatment on the basis of information adequate to make an informed decision is the standard. A decision on the part of one who provides health care to act in the best interests of the person may not override the decision of a patient able to make competent choices. The patient may choose between kinds of treatment on the basis of adequate information, or she may choose to forgo treatment. For the incompetent person, a guardian chooses on the basis of what that person believes to be in the best interests of the patient. Or the guardian suggests what he believes the patient would have decided if competent. Normally the decision maker will be a family group, usually the next of kin.

3. *Be honest.* That the physician and members of a patient's family should communicate honestly about the patient's diagnosis and the probable course of the disease is generally accepted. It was not always so. Fifty years ago, the physician or family frequently withheld information from a patient if they believed such information would be harmful. There were always problems of dishonesty. If the physician and family knew the patient had a life-threatening illness that was in its terminal stage and did not reveal it, the patient had no basis for planning and executing final acts. If the patients knew the disease was more serious than they were told, they probably felt worse and increasingly came to distrust the word of the physician and family.

Some would say there is a moral difference between actual lying and deceiving through withholding information. Loving care and concern may suggest limiting the amount of information that the patient receives. Relative honesty now is the standard; but more needs to be done in providing relevant medical information that will help them to understand their illnesses. This will promote the patient's role as autonomous partner in the processes of living and dying. Honesty seems integral to being truly human and to participating in covenant relationships such as those between the dying and their caretakers.

4. *Avoid killing.* Perhaps the most stringent of all moral pro-

hibitions is against taking life. The question of killing arises in every discussion of prolonging living and dying. If there are any conditions under which a newborn would be let die because there is no hope, we might ask whether it is not then rational to actively hasten such death—for example, to avoid slow starvation or a slow and painful death from cystic fibrosis. Or, when there is no hope of improvement for a person suffering from terminal cancer, would it be kinder, more merciful, and more humane to use an active means to end the suffering?

But to participate actively in terminating life is contrary to what patients and the family can rightfully expect of the professional who is committed to saving life. Some ethicists argue that the principle prohibiting killing should always hold because absolute certainty of either diagnosis or the future course of the disease is never possible. Some people who should die from a given condition continue to live. Even though there may be "mercy killings" that seem justifiable, the effects of permitting them are permanent and irreversible for the individual and may have long-term undesirable social consequences.

Others would say that killing another human being interrupts a life given by God and therefore takes into human hands what rightfully belongs only to God. Some ethicists believe that decisions to let persons die are morally quite different from acts intended to bring death. Many will find it not difficult to acquiesce in the first but impossible to concur with the second.

5. *Do justice.* Is it just to prolong an infant's life at great expense for a maximum of twelve months when those same funds could have saved many more lives? If saving a child's life results in ongoing pain and frustration for the child and the family, is it just to use the resources in that way when the same money could be used to provide a significantly higher quality of life for other candidates? Is it just to spend hundreds of thousands of dollars on artificial heart operations for twelve or eighteen months of life that is very limited when the same resources might be used in research or education that would prevent heart disease, making the artificial heart unnecessary?

These are the kinds of questions concerning justice that we must face. Four approaches people use to work through them:

(a) A just decision provides the most net benefit to the most persons. Those who use this approach place positive and negative values on the results of the possible course of action and let the decision regarding justice depend on striking a net balance.

(b) All persons are entitled to what they possess by the natural distribution of health characteristics and to what means they can purchase to enhance their health by work, trade, and income from other sources. Justice requires that the society protect all persons from the unjust or illegal appropriation of their possession of health and the means to enhance health.

(c) Justice requires that a society use its resources to secure the maximum welfare of those with minimal endowment. This approach would always result in giving priority to those with the greatest need.

(d) Justice provides for such treatment that the net welfare of all persons is equal. Some persons argue that all persons should have equal treatment. But can there be equal treatment if persons have very unequal needs and endowments at the beginning? This approach insists on the net welfare, thus taking into account the point at which the person begins as a result of the natural distribution.

Although these principles and approaches may yield the same result, many times they will conflict. Then it becomes clear that it is our view of life that really determines our decision.

What Is Your View of Human Life?

Some theologians say that life has *absolute* value because it is God's gift: "Then the Lord God formed man of dust from the ground, and breathed into his nostrils the breath of life; and man became a living being" (Genesis 2:7). Others would say that the fact that human life is called into being by God points to the *transcendence of God*. To assign *absolute* value to human life tends toward idolatry.

Some say that the source of value of human life is that humans are valuing creatures. Because they are of great value, we should terminate human life only with great reluctance and only for strongly overriding reasons. Others hold that "value language" is a trap. To speak of human life as having value obscures the essential nature of the human being. They prefer to speak of *the sanctity of human life.*

In this view life, the operative verbs would be *love, respect,* and *reverence.* The implications of this view are wrapped up in the statement, "Do not act or fail to act to *cause* someone's death." However, though one would never act intending the death of another, one might refrain from treatment to permit a person to complete the dying process. Because the dying process *can* be stopped does not necessarily mean that it *should* be stopped. We can love, respect, and reverence persons both in prolonging living and in permitting dying.

Yet another view that affects decision-making is that as Christians we are people of the resurrection. There is no fear of death because in Christ God has conquered death. Beyond death is life. Therefore, we do not have to hold onto life at any cost. At the appropriate time we can surrender it, looking forward to an eternity with God.

What Place Has the Church in These Questions?

For Christians, faith celebrated in worship and relationships cultivated through the faith fellowship may be most significant in dealing with the questions we have been thinking about. These issues are some of the most agonizing that we face. How may I be sure that my answers are acceptable to other thoughtful people with similar views regarding life and with like commitments? How can I be sure that when through my agony I have reached a decision, I will not be standing alone outside the moral consensus? The community of faith can and should provide assistance.

1. *Through study and discussion of the issues.* Study of the issues with a book like this one provides a basis for discussion within a group of ten to fifteen. It is not necessary for all to come to agreement; and certainly there should be no attempt to coerce agreement. To anticipate the scope of questions that one may face in medical crises, to come to some realization of responsibility for making decisions, to be aware of principles for decision-making, to clarify one's own view of human life—these are focuses for study and discussion. Those who participate in such studies are likely to face life's tough questions with a bit more balance and less panic

than had they never talked about these issues with others in the community of faith.

2. *Through providing support groups and persons.* No person or family should have to stand alone in the decision about whether to preserve the life of a baby who is fatally malformed. No family of father and grown children should need to be alone in the decision about whether and when to stop treatment of a mother for whom there is now no hope of cure. Not only do they need love and caring at these times; they also need assurance that their thoughts and judgments are truly consistent with the values of at least a significant portion of the community.

3. *Through celebrating living and dying.* Through its liturgy, however elaborate or simple, the church can assist the individual and the family in celebrating the passages of life by putting into words their spiritual meaning. Thus living and dying become of one piece—all of it holy.

For Discussion

Reread the two brief cases at the beginning of the chapter. Try to put yourself in the position of the different persons. Then answer the following questions.

1. If you were John and Leah, would you rush the baby to the city medical center to begin a series of attempts to save the baby?

2. Would you authorize the physician to let the baby die— perhaps only giving sedatives and feeding only on demand?

3. With whom would you want to talk in addition to your doctor?

4. If you were members of a support group in the church with John and Leah, what issues would you try to help them face?

5. Who would you side with in Steve and Eleanor's case— Steve or Eleanor's children? Why?

6. What kind of conversation should be taking place between Steve and Eleanor's doctor? What other conversations might be helpful to Steve?

7. How might the church be most helpful to Steve and Eleanor in this time?

8

Procreation: Extraordinary Means

Anne Krabill Hershberger

HUMAN REPRODUCTION used to seem so simple and predictable. A man and woman married, engaged in sexual intercourse, and very often a pregnancy followed. Usually after nine months, a healthy baby was born. Some babies were not healthy, and they often died shortly after birth. Some couples could not become parents through sexual intercourse; so their options were to try to adopt a child or remain childless.

Today the options have expanded. One can become a parent without marriage or a sexual partner. One can be sexually active and still avoid pregnancy, birth, and parenthood. During a woman's pregnancy, physicians sometimes can determine whether the baby will be healthy; and up to a certain time in the pregnancy, the parents can choose to end the pregnancy legally.

When a couple is infertile, one member of the couple can contribute sperm or ova to meet a third person's complementary sex cell to produce a baby. The male and female sex cells can meet in a petri dish and be put back into the mother's uterus or into another woman's uterus to complete the pregnancy. Additionally, scientists are trying to develop a process known as *ectogenesis*, or pregnancy outside the uterus. Unfortunately, all of this scientific "progress" has developed faster than our ability to adequately deal with the ethical dilemmas this new technology creates.

In this chapter I will (1) describe some of the reproductive technologies in use today—their ethical, social, psychological, and legal implications; (2) identify the biblical concepts that can inform us in analyzing and choosing alternatives; and (3) encourage personal and congregational involvement in decision-making in relation to that technology.

Artificial Insemination by Donor

When a couple experiences the pain of infertility, as do one out of six married couples in the United States, or when people fear transmitting a genetically induced disease to their offspring, *collaborative reproductive techniques* can become attractive options. These techniques require the participation (collaboration) of a third person so that a man and woman may produce a child, as in artificial insemination by donor (AID) or surrogate motherhood. In AID, a physician uses a syringe to deposit a donor's sperm into the wife's uterus during her time of ovulation. Up to 20,000 children conceived in this way are born in the United States each year.

In the surrogate mother procedure, a couple enters a contract with a woman outside the marriage to undergo artificial insemination using the husband's sperm. She carries and bears his child. Then at birth, or soon after, she gives up all parental rights and transfers physical custody of the child to the couple for adoption by the wife.

Whatever the method, collaborative reproduction raises many legal, social, psychological, and ethical questions. From a legal perspective: Does it constitute adultery? What is the legitimacy status of the resulting child in respect to claims on inheritance, child support, custody, and visitation privileges if the couple should divorce? What is the legal liability of the physician who screened and matched the donor or surrogate to the couple?

More psychological and social questions arise. Will the couple be able to cope with their unequal biological relationship to the child (only one contributed genetically to the child)? What are the ramifications of the child's inability to know half of his or her genetic-medical history? Might the child marry a close biological relative unknowingly? In the case of AID, the wife may long to meet the man who "helped" her when her husband could not. Might the husband's inability to sire a child threaten his masculinity? Could it cause him to develop a sense of inadequacy in relation to other men or cause him to withdraw from the home and seek self-fulfillment elsewhere? If the couple is endangered psychologically, the child may feel alienation from the father and suffer psychologically as well.

The ethical issues inherent in collaborative reproduction stem from our belief about the nature and meaning of marriage and parenthood. What is the proper relationship between the marriage bond and the procreation of children? Some would argue that since the donor and surrogate develop no deeply personal relationship, this technique poses no questions of infidelity for the husband and wife if they agree to have children by this means. However, others would argue that the marriage bond and procreation are inseparable. It is not that married couples must have children, but that they must not procreate from beyond their marriage.

For all the parties involved in collaborative reproduction, difficult issues are present. For the infertile couple, collaborative reproduction may involve procreation outside the marriage. For the donors of sperm and the surrogate mothers, procreation is reduced to the status of a service for hire (or donation). They are encouraged to distance themselves from their offspring and their own bodies. There is no loving commitment to the child's other parent, and they have no intention of caring for the children they deliberately share in conceiving. To justify a decision to become a donor of sperm or a surrogate mother, some say they wanted to provide the gift of life and help a childless couple. This is commendable; but are there not limits to one's altruism?

It is difficult to assess the effects of collaborative reproduction on the potential child, for without the cooperation of the infertile couple and the third party, the child would never exist; but no one argues that all potential children ought to exist. The chief issues for a child conceived technologically center on a confused or nonexistent relationship with his or her one biological parent. One should consider the potential psychological damage that results from deceiving the child about his or her unusual origins. Or if the child knows this, does he or she sense the rejection by the parent who deliberately planned never to care for the child or who was paid to bring about his or her being?

The above discussion centers on the more usual situation of those requesting the services of a donor of sperm or a surrogate mother—the infertile married couple. There are other situations that cause people to seek these services and that raise further ethical issues: single people with no sexual partner who desire to parent their own children, gay couples who want children, and the use of third parties who are known to the couple needing their help.

An important basic question that society, and particularly Christians, should ask in light of these dilemmas is this: Just because collaborative reproduction works, do we have to use it? From the standpoint of ethics, we need to be concerned both about right ends and right means.

In Vitro Fertilization

Other reproductive technologies that raise ethical issues are in vitro fertilization (IVF) and embryo transfer. The procedure for IVF and embryo transfer was first developed in England when doctors surgically removed an ovum from Lesley Brown's ovary and fertilized it with her husband's sperm in a petri dish. The doctors performed this procedure because Mrs. Brown's fallopian tubes were blocked and her ova could not reach the tubes and uterus for fertilization and implantation. Three days later doctors implanted the fertilized ovum into her uterus and her pregnancy proceeded normally. Louise Joy Brown was born 25 July, 1978—the first test-tube baby. Estimates of the number of couples who could potentially benefit from IVF in the United States range between 450,000 and 600,000.

The main purpose of IVF today is to enable infertile couples to have a child conceived of their own sex cells when the infertility problem stems from blockage of the female's fallopian tubes. (IVF also can use ova from the wife or a donor and the fertilized ova can be implanted in the wife or a surrogate mother.) However, other possible applications of IVF include the establishment of embryo banks, use of frozen embryos in research, transfer of embryos to a surrogate mother, screening of embryos for specific chromosomal characteristics or defects (sex, genetic disease).

IVF has a 20 percent success rate in bringing about viable pregnancies. This is similar to the success rate for normal intercourse. Issues that often arise, however, in analyzing the appropriateness of using IVF include the artificiality of the procedure, the question of embryo wastage, the possibility of endangering the prospective child, and the problem of containment.

Some Christians believe that there should be no separation of sexual union and reproduction. IVF, however, does not inherently need to depend on a third person, as does AID or surrogate motherhood. Therefore this procedure does not necessarily jeopardize the marriage relationship. If the artificiality of IVF is an issue, then Christians would need to question their use of eyeglasses or pacemakers as well.

In the laboratory work associated with IVF, some fertilized ova are destroyed or wasted through manipulation, some because they seem abnormal, and some for the sake of research. So again there are questions. Does this treatment for a specific type of infertility justify destruction of some early embryos? What happens to the frozen embryos that are not implanted, that have no chance for future life? The embryos that are implanted or frozen or wasted would not be present except in the interests of human life. Some of them will not have a chance at life; but without them, none would have that chance.

The concern that IVF could cause defective babies is apparently not founded. Research indicates that the incidence of abnormal babies is no greater among those conceived by IVF than among those conceived naturally.

The question of containment raises the *slippery slope* issue—what will the procedure lead to? We must remember that all decisions in life place us on a slippery slope. We can go to extremes on any issue. Will our society be prudent enough to allow IVF to be the very helpful technique it can be in assisting infertile couples; or will the temptation to use IVF to genetically influence future generations, for example, put a moral cloud on its use?

Another very real social issue related to IVF and its containment is the matter of priorities. Should a couple's desire for a child permit them or society to spend $4,000 per treatment, excluding doctor's fees, to engage in technological reproduction that may not be successful, while funds for basic health care, education, and good nutrition are not available for thousands of children already born?

Even if Christians agree that IVF is morally neutral, some future procedures that rely on the IVF technique may pose moral dilemmas. One such procedure is surrogate embryo transfer. This is the insertion of a fertilized ovum into the uterus of a woman who did not provide the ovum. Another procedure is ova and embryo banking or stockpiling frozen ova and fertilized ova.

Embryo transfer with ova or embryo banking could be used in these situations as well: (1) A woman with healthy ovaries but with uterine disease or no uterus could use her own ova, fertilize them, and then transfer them to another's uterus. The woman carrying the pregnancy in this case would be a genuine surrogate. (2) A woman with a healthy uterus who did not want to use her own ova (perhaps because of fear of passing on a genetically induced disease) could use another woman's ova, fertilize them with her husband's sperm artificially, and transfer the resulting embryo to her own uterus or implant a frozen embryo formed from neither partner's sex cells. In the latter case, the embryo bank provides for a "very early adoption" possibility.

Many people believe that IVF used within certain guidelines, like using only the sex cells of a husband and wife, presents no ethical problems. This technology could be a real benefit for couples who struggle with infertility. However, the reproductive technologies like embryo transfer to surrogates and embryo banking that depend upon IVF can potentially raise ethical issues like the deliberate creation of human life not desired by either genetic parent, or some of the legal, social, psychological, and ethical issues raised earlier in relation to AID and surrogate motherhood.

More commonplace reproductive technology might include the area of contraception. Although many Christians can morally justify and, indeed, feel a responsibility to use natural, mechanical, or chemical means of contraception, there are situations even for these people when contraceptive use is questionable. There is a case in point.

Sandy, a sixteen-year-old high school sophomore, entered the school nurse's office obviously under stress. They had developed a good relationship prior to this, but now Sandy refused to look at the nurse while she spoke. After a period of careful questioning and listening, the nurse uncovered Sandy's reason for coming. She wanted information about birth control and where to get it. The nurse was a Christian woman who clearly wanted to help this distressed young woman, but what constituted help in this case?

This kind of request put the nurse in an awkward position. One can assume that a decision to be sexually active preceded this request. It is praiseworthy that Sandy attempted to be responsible about avoiding parenthood as a single person; but obviously the concern about avoiding parenthood could have been removed by abstaining from sexual intercourse. Does one condone premarital sexual intercourse by providing birth-control information to unmarried people? What else did Sandy really need from the nurse?

Possible Christian Responses

How should we as Christians respond to technological reproduction? Some Christians will say, "Stay clear of these new technologies. We ought not to play God." Other Christians see these developments as part of God revealing his creation to us and that we are to have dominion over it.

The Bible obviously does not provide a tailor-made Christian response to AID, surrogate motherhood (except in the story of Abraham, Sarah, and Hagar), IVF, embryo transfer or contraception. However, as James Burtness points out, "There are ... implications of biblical faith that may help to inform possible responses to the ethical issues raised by the debate" (*Questions about the Beginning of Life,* ed. Edward Schneider [Augsburg Publishing House, 1985], p. 89).

(1) The Christian outlook should point toward optimism rather than pessimism, expecting good rather than bad results from new discoveries. The Christian ought never to be frozen into inaction because of the presence of risks or the absence of complete data. Christians know it is impossible to do anything without making some mistakes.

(2) Because the outlook of the church is characteristically full of hope, its expectations of the future ought to, and often do, feed back into the making of current decisions.

(3) The Christian who operates from a stance of hopefulness, believing that God is working through human history and through the history of nature, will be inclined to place the burden of proof on those who oppose a given type of scientific research.

(4) The Christian knows that God created everything through and for Christ. There is therefore no need to fear new information about anything.

(5) Because of its confidence in the redemptive possibilities of human activity, the church will tend to think that regulation is possible. Because of its awareness of the demonic potential of human activity, it will insist that regulation is necessary.

If new procedures such as IVF appear to be full of promise, the tendency ought to be toward investigating the possibilities. Are we in danger of playing God? Not really; for this technological method only builds on the prior divine gift of human reproduction.

The Bible does give guidance regarding the relative importance of procreation and parenthood for those in God's covenant community. The Bible message is that the family is to be held in great esteem with God's blessing. He commands that parents are to be honored, children are to be celebrated as gifts from God, the capacity to procreate through loving intercourse is to be cherished, and that grief should be acknowledged when natural procreation is not possible. An even stronger message from the Bible that is pertinent to the subject of this chapter is that the family is not the only or even the most important dimension of human life. Covenant faith with God is.

The kinds of questions raised by reproductive technologies are questions that Christians should not need to face alone. The use of reproductive technologies present an uncharted course for most people. How helpful Christians could be to each other if together they could gather information about the suggested technology to be used or decisions being faced, share their thoughts on what the inherent issues are, study the related biblical principles, identify alternative courses of action, and together pray for guidance to help the persons directly involved to decide in the best way possible.

If Sandy's nurse had anticipated the kind of request that Sandy presented and had sought help in thinking through it with Christian friends prior to the encounter, she likely would have brought to the situation a good understanding of the magnitude of the problems associated with teenage sexuality and pregnancy. She would have gained a knowledge of resources in the community and church to help youth think through their lifestyle choices and had greater confidence in the approach she used. She would know after careful discernment that Christian friends supported her in this and, yes, had the ability to educate Sandy in areas of needed help.

Most Christians would likely agree that children are wonderful gifts entrusted by God, but they are not gifts to be sought at any price. Costs to the integrity of the marriage, to the personhood of all involved, and to the resulting child may be too high in some instances. May God grant us the good sense to recognize the complexity of the issues surrounding reproductive technologies and a sincere love for our brothers and sisters to discern together what seems to be the best possible decisions given our imperfect vision.

For Discussion

1. If faced with a long-standing infertility problem and a strong desire for your own children, what technological options would you consider appropriate?

2. If a friend in the family of faith chooses to use a reproductive technique that you personally cannot accept as appropriate for a Christian, how would you respond to that friend?

3. What kind of response from the school nurse would be most loving and helpful to Sandy? To her potential children?

9

Organ Transplants

Myron Ebersole

ERMA YOUNG, a married woman in her early thirties, developed kidney stones, which eventually led to serious kidney disease. Despite aggressive treatment, she developed end-stage renal disease—kidney failure from which there is no expectation of recovery. Erma than began hemodialysis at a nearby hospital center twice a week for four hours each day. Though the treatment saved her life, she felt sick and had severely decreased appetite and energy so that she was unable to continue her work in the family business. Three years after beginning dialysis, she came to a university medical center for evaluation for a kidney transplant. A few months after the assessment, a kidney became available that matched her blood and tissue types.

Within a short time, Erma was able to resume her work in the family business. Receiving a transplant and the return to normalcy were a profoundly religious experience for her. She feels that through the gift of the kidney and the work of all the medical staff, her life has been transformed. She now appears with transplant-team personnel in public presentations, gives talks at dialysis centers to encourage patients who are considering transplantation, and speaks in behalf of the Kidney-One organ donor foundation. "God has so richly blessed me that I must do all I can to help others. It is my way of repaying all that I have been given," she says.

■ ■ ■

Late one night the Miller family was called to the hospital. There a doctor told them that their son Brian had been in an auto accident. He had sustained a severe blow to his head and might well be brain dead. As they waited for a definitive diagnosis, they visited Brian, an athletic handsome nineteen-year-old. He seemed to be lying quietly and peacefully as though sleeping—except for the respirator. The doctor suggested that the Millers might want to consider donating Brian's organs to retrieve some meaning from the tragedy. Their first reaction was a very clear refusal. They had not yet been able to accept Brian's death. Mr. Miller insisted that they take every measure to save his life.

The neurosurgeons carefully evaluated their tests for brain death and concluded that Brian was indeed dead. He was unresponsive to any stimuli; the electroencephalogram showed no brain activity; and when the respirator was removed, his breathing stopped. When the doctors repeated the tests twenty-four hours later, the family was forced to accept the diagnosis of brain death. However, still holding on to one last hope, Mr. Miller requested to be present when they removed the respirator so that he could see the body stop breathing on its own and finally be convinced. As he sadly turned away, he asked that Brian be anesthetized for the operation to remove the organs so that he would not suffer any pain.

■ ■ ■

Transplant technology is not yet perfected. It has transformed many lives from certain early death to vibrant productivity. Others have had their hopes raised only to experience the inability of the transplant to stem the inevitable course of organ failure and death. Medicine has taken giant steps forward in its ability to alter the course of life for many and to stimulate fantasies about prolonged life. But it has also raised ethical, theological, social, economic, and political issues.

In the face of uncertain results, limited resources, and high costs, institutions have pressed forward to establish more and more programs. Although only three institutions were doing liver transplants in 1981, 34 were doing them in 1986. Only five performed heart transplants in 1981; in 1986 there were 58.

The number of procedures also is rising. From 62 hearts transplanted in 1981, transplants in the United States rose to 346 in 1984. Liver transplants rose from 26 to 308; and kidney transplants from 4,885 to 6,968 in the same period.

Survival rates are also improving rapidly. The one-year survival rate for heart recipients has reached 80 percent; for liver recipients, 65 to 70 percent; for kidney recipients, over 90 percent (Jeff Lyon, "Organ Transplants: Conundra Without End," *Second Opinion* 1 [March 1986]: 43-44). Behind these statistics are improved survival and tissue-matching techniques and a greatly increased ability to deal with the problems of immunology, especially through immunosuppressant drugs. Thus, the highly risky transplant procedures are much more reliable.

But what are the questions? Is this not an outstanding example of the successes of modern science? In an article "Organ Transplantation: The Costs of Success," Arthur L. Caplan writes that the moral problems that relate to organ transplants include: (1) the inadequate supply of organs and the problem of equitable distribution, (2) the high costs of transplantation, and (3) the lack of adequate government control over transplant programs (*The Hastings Center Report* [December 1983]: 23-32). To these we must add the problem of investing limited health care dollars in this form of treatment to the neglect of other forms of treatment, illness prevention, and health promotion.

In this chapter, I will focus primarily on the issue of procuring organs for transplants. Particularly I will consider why the significant shortfall in available organs and how we might move to resolve this problem.

Organ Procurement

The supply of organs has been falling far short of demand. At any given time in the United States there are some 100 people in need of donor hearts; 300 waiting for livers; 30 for pancreases; and 8,000 for kidneys. Because the organ retrieval and transplantation system is still in its early stages, it is probable that many who would otherwise be suitable recipients are never worked up for transplantation. This is more likely for those who need organs other than kidneys. (Kidney failure is treatable by renal dialysis, enabling the potential kidney recipient to wait much longer until a suitable kidney is available. And since only one kidney is necessary, needs are met twice as rapidly as the need for other organs. Further, living related donors—parents and siblings—who can give one kidney and live satisfactorily with the remaining one often provide the needed organ.)

In institutions that perform transplants, it is common to see examples of the dramatic and anxious waiting that sometimes has a tragic outcome. After months of waiting, the hospital may call a recipient because an organ is apparently available—perhaps hundreds of miles away—only to find out that last-minute tissue matching indicates that the organ is not suitable. Some patients are uneasily aware that during bad weather they wonder whether there will be more accidents, thus making more organs available.

More troubling, however, is the persistent resistance to donate organs. While 94 percent of the people in a national sample of 2,056 were aware of organ transplantation, only 19 percent had signed donor cards. The survey showed that 53 percent would agree to donate the organs of a relative who had just died, while 50 percent would donate their own organs (Manninea and Evans, "Public Attitudes and Behavior Regarding Organ Donation," *Journal of the American Medical Association* 253 [7 June 1985]: 3111-15). A Gallup poll reported in the *New York Times*, 3 May, 1987, noted that 82 percent of the respondents would donate adult relatives' organs; 61 percent would give permission if the donor was their child; and 48 percent would donate their own organs. However, only 20 percent had completed a donor card.

Problems of organ donation are not related to personal reactions alone. The criteria for brain death, alluded to above in the case of Brian, have grown out of medical and legal needs resulting from the increasing life-support capabilities of medical technology. The cessation of heart function and breathing, long the signs for defining death, is no longer adequate. Now we can maintain bodily functions despite irreversible brain injuries. The resulting dilemma for families, including the massive economic costs, led to the Uniform Determination of Death Act of 1981. According to this statute, a person may be declared dead if there is irreversible cessation of the entire brain, including the brain stem, which controls autonomic bodily functions. Virtually all of the states in the United States have brain-death laws based on this concept. This development came at an opportune time for organ retrieval and transplantation.

There are still those who fear that brain-death criteria will be used to justify early pronouncement of death to procure organs for others. "In his book *The Way We Die*, David Dempsey writes: 'Once [the physician] is satisfied that the brain has died . . . his incentive to prolong life is diminished. Thus what began as heroic medicine, in the gallant sense of the word, threatens to become a device to regulate the death of one person for the benefit of another' " (Lyon, p. 51).

Others argue that brain death is not the same as true death and that the declaration of death on the basis of such criteria represents *prognosis* rather than *diagnosis*. It presumes to speak what only God can decide. Neither physicians nor families have a right to donate another's organs. However, a person could decide that under the conditions of true death, one's body and organs could be used for research or transplantation—a decision one can only make for oneself (Lyon, p. 53).

Mainline Catholic thought, as well as most Protestant and Jewish groups, have accepted brain death—along with other responsible scientific criteria—as the basis for decisions about death. However, certain fundamentalist sects hold that complete bodily integrity is essential to assure resurrection of the body. Orthodox Judaism also resists organ donation on the basis of brain-death criteria, based on the belief that life is determined by the presence of breath—this despite their approval in theory of organ donation that would save the life of another.

Other issues that complicate organ donation include: (1) fears of family members that they will not be able to have a normal funeral with viewing; (2) arbitrary refusal to consider the request for organs, sometimes even in the face of the wishes of the deceased; (3)

decisions of organ-procurement personnel to avoid obvious stress for the family; (4) the occasional anger or frustration by family members over the loss of a loved one expressed as resentment and resistance to any further involvement with medical activity, at least at the moment they are faced with such a request.

For several years it has been recognized that a primary reason for the failure to procure transplantable organs has been the reticence and even refusal of medical personnel to ask the family for the donation. For some it seems an admission of failure in medical treatment. Others fear legal repercussions. Still others fear it may interfere with the family's trust of their physician's commitment to care. Recently a number of states have passed *mandatory request laws*, which require that families be asked to donate their loved ones' organs in every case of death in which there are retrievable organs of any kind. The requirement by law would justify the physician's making the request despite the above possible objections.

Some have suggested the adoption of *presumed consent laws*, which allow organs to be removed routinely unless specific objections are expressed by a card carried by the individual or by members of the family. Critics contend that this policy would be too coercive and might infringe upon the rights of religious minorities who contend that any postmortem operations are mutilations of the dead body (Caplan, p. 23). Such laws, already on the books in France, have been essentially ignored because of moral reservations by hospital staff.

The American transplant system has relied upon voluntary giving and informed consent to provide needed organs. It has become evident that this does not assure that adults (or minors) who could do so are, in fact, providing an adequate supply. Thus, a policy of *encouraged voluntarism* has developed. Many ethicists, as well as the American Council on Transplantation, have supported this.

Critics have objected to the cost of the efforts to make encouraged voluntarism effective. And the fact that relatively few brain-dead victims have shown up in hospital emergency rooms with donor cards has raised serious questions among many about the adequacy of this approach. They also fear that it may contribute to developing a commercial market for the selling of organs. The last option has been essentially ruled out by legislation prohibiting the sale of organs.

Public policy, especially with the Uniform Anatomical Gift Act of 1968, has decided in favor of encouraged voluntarism. It has recognized the validity of living wills and organ-donor cards, along with the right of next of kin to make decisions regarding the donations of bodies or body parts. However, some claim that encouraged voluntarism is failing, since the supply of organs has remained fairly stable overall for several years. Massive educational efforts have apparently served well to *inform* the public but not to *motivate* significant change in the numbers of those who indicate readiness to donate their organs by signing and carrying organ-donor cards. Mandatory request laws are still so new that a significant trend is not yet evident.

Inasmuch as encouraged voluntarism, based on public education, has not met the need, is there an alternative? Significant change in the motivation to donate may be dependent on the religious communities. It may be that the church is best able to institute an educational program that will enable people to deal with their aversion to the retrieval process, including the invasion of the body after death. Significant change in attitudes is more likely to occur as people are given opportunity to explore their feelings and convictions with a trusted group.

It should be possible for the church to move beyond *informational education* about organ donation and transplantation to *transformational education* in relation to attitudes, feelings, and motivation. Such an education-transformation process would be able to help people: (1) find personally satisfying answers to questions about the morality of invasive procedures into the body after death; (2) resolve feelings of aversion and enable development of new attitudes toward organ retrieval; (3) deal with questions about the effects of such procedures in relation to life after death; and (4) develop motivational support for a stewardship and life-giving point of view.

Other Ethical Questions

The discussion of organ donation and retrieval points toward the question of patient selection. Health policy is increasingly public policy. Thus, donated organs have become public resources rather than private gifts. Transplantation professionals have become trustees or stewards of these organs in behalf of the community rather than mere private practitioners. The criteria for deciding who gets the organs must be fair to all.

Implementing a policy of fairness depends on various factors. On strictly medical grounds, decisions would be based on the determination of need and the probability that the recipient would benefit from the transplanted organ. These criteria reflect a concern for optimal benefit to patients who suffer from end-stage organ failure. A further medical concern is the relationship between urgency of need and probability of success. Thus a choice between two patients, both of whom urgently need transplants to survive, will likely favor the one for whom the transplant is most likely to succeed—hardly a fair choice for the one who loses. That loss is the dilemma the medical community faces, knowing that each year thousands die while waiting for organs that could be transplanted if they were given by families at the time of a loved one's death.

A first-come-first-served policy among patients who are equally good candidates may be quite satisfactory until other factors enter in. For example, how should age impact decision-making? Should an 18-year-old have preference over a 55-year-old? Many would say 55-year-olds have had their lives while 18-year-olds deserve a chance to fulfill their potentialities. However, would the choice change if the 18-year-old were a member of a motorcycle gang and on drugs while the 55-year-old were a respected teacher?

How should we make decisions where lifestyle is a probable cause of the problem? Should we favor a person who has had previous transplants, the last of which is failing, over one who has never received a transplant? Should welfare patients receive donated organs, or only those who can pay? What if the welfare patient is a mother of several children under twelve and the person who can pay is a single physician with a promising career? Should transplant candidates from the area where the organs were retrieved have priority for those organs? Should nonimmigrant aliens who are able to pay receive transplants in this country? Or what if the alien is a young and very talented person with little money? On what basis could a Christian favor excluding such applicants?

Finally, how should transplantations be paid for? The options are fairly well known: private pay; government funding through Medicare, Medicaid, or special appropriations; health insurance; and private fund drives for individual organ recipients. Each of these sources has effects on the resources available for other health care activities, including health promotion and disease prevention. Consider also the implications of the trend of increasing numbers of major organ transplants coupled with the high cost of each procedure. What is just?

How Does the Christian Decide?

Christians are responsible as individuals, as family members, as members of the Christian church—local congregation, denomination, and the church universal—and as citizens of their countries to be involved in making decisions about organ donation and transplantation. The values of a secular and materialistic society that promote self-sufficiency are sometimes distorted to such a degree that people are indifferent to the needs of others, as seen in the resistance to organ donation cited above. Materialistic values, anxiety about the body as representation of the loved family member, and an overemphasis on the resurrection of the physical body also contribute to refusal to consider organ donation.

As Christians who are members of the church consider these issues, they will need to reexamine the sources of their values by studying the biblical understandings of the body and the values of their particular Christian community. They will need to recognize that organ donation and transplantation represent more than remarkable advances of medical technology. They also represent opportunities to extend meaningful life to people in need. Organ donation can be a significant way of continuing in partnership with our Creator in the life process. It can be an act of compassion, of loving stewardship of our bodies. Alleviating suffering while serving others—both in life and death—is an expression of Christlike loving.

For Discussion

1. How do you feel about the transplantation of organs to save or enhance another person's life? What would be your wish if some-

one in your family needed an organ transplant?

2. Who should be the primary beneficiaries of transplant technology? What criteria should determine who gets available organs? How important should ability to pay be in making this decision?

3. Have you signed an organ-donor card? If not, why not? Is it partly because you haven't taken the time to think about the issue? If so, what types of information do you need to help you make an informed decision? How might you obtain this information?

4. What do you believe about the resurrection of persons? How has this belief influenced your attitudes toward donating your organs for transplant? If necessary, spend some time looking at what the Scriptures say about the body and resurrection. You might use a concordance, a topical Bible, or a Bible dictionary.

5. How do you respond to this statement: Donating organs can be a primary act of Christian loving and stewardship.

10

Genetic Engineering

Paul W. Hoffman

IN EARLY 1980, there was a controversial attempt by American medical personnel to replace defective hemoglobin genes in the bone marrow of patients in Italy and Israel. The experiments were done there because the Institutional Review Board (IRB) of the researchers' home institution, the University of California at Los Angeles, wanted them to do more animal experiments before experimenting on humans. The researchers replied that experimental attempts at gene therapy were the only hope for patients with fatal disorders like beta thalassemia, a severe anemia arising from an inherited hemoglobin abnormality. . . .

Genetic engineering is a powerful new medical technology. Its actual accomplishments so far are primitive, compared with expected developments. Because it manipulates the most fundamental elements of organic life, genes, in much the same way that nuclear physicists manipulate atoms, serious and legitimate concerns have been raised about present and future developments. Clearly there are risks. Experimentation on human beings is a necessary phase in the successful development of any new medical technology. A few individuals and families will face the dilemma of deciding whether to take the risk. The society at large has produced rules ... for experimentation on human subjects. ... What risks connected with genetic engineering are we willing to accept? How can we responsibly control such necessary and inevitable risks? (From Frank Harron, John Burnside, MD., and Tom Beauchamp, *Health and Human Values: A Guide to Making Your Own Decisions* [New Haven: Yale University Press, 1983], pp. 175-77.)

■ ■ ■

The understanding of DNA (deoxyribonucleic acid), the building blocks of life, in terms of its impact on genetic characteristics began about 1953. It was in the early 1970s that scientists learned how to isolate specific DNA materials and remove them from one species and attach them to another. Scientists coined the term *genetic engineering* in 1965. But the rapid changes in genetic engineering really began in 1980.

An era often comes upon us and is gone before we label or identify it. We are currently in the *genetic era*, likely the most powerful era of all times in terms of the potential for major changes. This era will quickly outdistance the impact of the computer revolution and presents exciting, different, promising, and frightening scientific achievements.

Science and religion both seek to improve the human experience. From time to time their different procedures and values have, by events, demanded conversation and cooperation. Such is the case now as persons experience living in the genetic era. The rapid changes in scientific technology have been exciting, frightening, different, and promising. Many in religious communities have become apprehensive, pensive, and concerned.

Some Current Challenges

The following are examples of what is happening and what will likely happen in the near future. In each case, Christians face the challenge of bringing their faith in Christ into a fundamental conversation with science. When facing real medical dilemmas, simplistic and exclusive declarations of faith—either in historic beliefs or in medical technology—probably will be inadequate.

One, our biotechnology is advancing and changing much more

rapidly than most have envisioned. Many of the genetic advances that were predicted in the early 1980s as being possibilities by 1990 or the turn of the century have already been realized. Scientific articles are susceptible to being outdated before they are printed. Within a very short time we have moved from viewing bacteria DNA on an X-ray photograph to trimming, clipping, and changing minute parts of the genetic code. So there are many things that we *can do*; and our technological capacities are ever increasing. The issue is discerning when we *should do* all that we can do. And how much further do we push out the technological frontiers while many in our world live without necessities?

Two, the process of reproduction is being expanded. The usual process of coitus, pregnancy, and birth is no longer always the procedure. New reproductive technologies involve in vitro fertilization, artificial insemination, and storage of both eggs and sperm for use at a later time. Single persons often become parents through conscious choices. Some women serve as surrogate mothers to provide an infant for childless persons. Some parents choose laboratory techniques to virtually assure the sex of their child. Chapter 8 points up some of the ethical challenges of developments in this area.

Three, the diagnosing of disease is rapidly moving away from an art form toward a precise science. There are few limits to what researchers foresee in the ability to detect genes in a fetus that might contribute to cancer, heart ailments, diabetes, hypertension, and more. Special diagnostic kits are now being developed for use by both physicians and laypersons. Some kits will now precisely diagnose mononucleosis and cytomegalovirus and can detect chlamydia, currently the most common venereal disease.

The ethical dilemmas involved in genetic screening are formidable. For example, sickle-cell anemia occurs primarily among blacks; Tay-Sachs disease is unique to persons of Jewish extraction; and one in every twenty Caucasians is a carrier of cystic fibrosis. Is it fair to screen particular races of persons or ethnic groups for a particular disease? Should such screening be mandatory? Who should have access to the results?

Four, genetic experiments are getting closer to involving human beings in major ways. Gene therapy involving animals is now fairly common. Some simple genetic changes will likely be made involving human beings in which unhealthy genes will be replaced by healthy ones. While genetic therapy involving somatic cells will be a first step, therapy involving germline cells is certainly not far away. Sickle-cell anemia, hemophilia, dwarfism, certain viruses, and cancer are examples of disease thought to be treatable through genetic technologies.

Five, many biotechnologists are becoming entrepreneurs. Traditionally, scientists have been viewed as scholars whose fulfillment has come through what has been called "pure" research. But genetic engineering is a multibillion-dollar business. In the race to be first with achievements, companies have paid very lucrative salaries to genetic scientists to become a part of their industries. Many are concerned that as scientists become entrepreneurs, motivated by business interests, the usual checks and balances or motivations for research that have been present in previous years may be lessened. Will profit become the prevailing ethic as we experiment with the basic building blocks of life?

Six, there is at present a lack of valid regulations for biotechnology. In August 1985, the heads of several United States federal government agencies accepted a proposal to create a new Biotechnology Science Board, which would have the authority over research and development in genetic engineering. There was much disagreement over this direction; and, as yet, nothing has happened. Thus there is no acceptable and adequate regulatory group for the technologies already in place. And there is no single agency that has the power to regulate genetic research. In the absence of any regulatory group asking fundamental ethical questions, will the consumer be at the mercy of the best salespersons?

Seven, the potential exists for changing the very form of human life. It is only a matter of time until the entire DNA sequence of human beings will be computerized and cataloged. The potential to change human life-forms is present in ways that are beyond our comprehension. The theological, sociological, and scientific questions that this raises are monumental, unavoidable, and not easily resolved. The changes immediately ahead may be more rapid, significant, and disturbing than we imagine. A simplicity of attitude or ignoring what is taking place is not an appropriate

Christian response. In addition to those mentioned above, here are other questions related to genetic engineering that Christians will have to face:

1. What does it mean to be created in God's image?

2. Is there a core of humanness that makes us the godlike creatures that we are? How would you describe that core?

3. Does manipulating the genetic code alter that core? If so, is it ethically permissible to tamper with the essence of humanity?

4. Is it possible to establish norms for human alterations that will be consistent with God's creation? What might such norms look like?

5. Who are the appropriate persons who should have the right to exercise power over the destiny of others?

6. What is the proper way for the Christian community to work with the scientific community in making decisions that are moral and appropriate?

7. What are the moral limits in genetic change beyond which it is sinful to go?

8. Is it socially responsible to give free reign to a biotechnological industry when the bottom line is profit?

9. Will positive genetic change for health reasons be available only to those with the resources to afford it?

10. What impact will genetic changes have on our ecological system, which has a delicate balance?

11. What impact will genetic engineering have on reproduction?

12. Ultimately, who will determine which biologically developed species are acceptable?

Congregations Get Involved

The questions above are very real and appropriate; future directions are not clear. Probably no single topic could be developed that would embody the issues that are of concern to Christians— life, death, birth, sickness, health, abortion, reproduction, hunger, right, wrong, creation, medicines, war, peace—as does genetic engineering. Thus, Christians will wisely take what is happening in biotechnology very seriously. The following are five areas that might be considered for immediate attention.

One, theologians—more specifically moral theologians—need to be involved in the decision-making processes related to genetic engineering. As science continues carefully to unravel DNA's double helix, as scientists continue to map out the essence of life, as viral diseases, cancer, and even certain aspects of the aging process become manageable and manipulable, it is imperative that the religious community develop statements and establish an equilibrium. The future needs to be determined by theologians, philosophers, and social scientists in addition to the scientists.

Two, special counseling seminars and classes to assist professional persons are essential. Pastors, physicians, biologists, psychologists, and others who do counseling with persons would profit from up-to-date information about biotechnology to be total counselors. At present, those involved in assisting with genetic issues are considered to be quite successful in providing medical information, but less than satisfactory in addressing the emotional, economic, and moral issues that are involved. Spiritual and compassionate advisers who have an initial understanding of the medical intricacies involved in genetics are needed now; and the need can only increase.

Three, it is most important that legislation and regulations be developed related to biotechnology. High priority should be given to establishing an appropriate legislative body or commission to regulate the research and procedures in genetic engineering. The procedures for such developments are unclear, but voters must speak. Coordinating planning is essential for the good of all. While the potential for good is great, the potential for harm to present and future generations is also present.

Four, entire congregations can appropriately become involved in discussing the ethical issues involved with genetic engineering. Christians, scientists and nonscientists, have a compassionate orientation that makes them especially equipped to determine what is good and what is bad in biotechnology. Appropriate safeguards are mandatory to prevent the use of the poor or uneducated in genetic research. It is questionable for academic institutions to promote or accept lucrative contracts when the sole purpose of the contracts is for research to produce weapons for military defense. Christians might consider ways to use the powerful genetic technologies to relieve human suffering in areas such as the third world and especially when the financial rewards are limited.

Five, the teaching ministry of the church can have an impact on local communities. A systematic method of presenting information through classes, forums, debates, and discussions within congregations may be one of our highest priorities for these days.

Conclusion

The advancements of genetic engineering have begun to provide us with choices in areas where previously no choices were possible. Existing moral and ethical systems do not always give clear guidelines for making these choices. We have crossed the barriers into the very essence of life. There is no going back. If we proceed deliberately and insist on guidelines that are subservient to the norm of love, it may be possible to have a future with increased joy and fulfillment as we place our faith in God to shape our ultimate destiny.

For Discussion

1. What are some of the potential benefits of genetic engineering? What are some of the possible misuses of this technology?

2. Imagine that a couple in your church wanted to have children but through gene screening, they knew that they had a high probability of producing children with a genetic disease. How would you counsel this couple? Suppose they decided to conceive a child and then through genetic testing of the fetus discovered that the child indeed had a genetic disease. What options would you present to them?

3. Should scientists try to eliminate genetic diseases through actually manipulating human genes or should they focus on screening and helping persons to act preventively?

4. If you have not done so, think about and discuss the questions on page 117.

11

Allocating Limited Medical Resources

Stan Godshall

NEAR THE BEGINNING of the present technology explosion in the early 1960s, the Swedish Hospital in Seattle, Washington, formed a "public committee" to decide who would have access to a scarce medical resource—the kidney machine. The discussions of this "God Committee" were public, and the debate raged about criteria for access to the machine. The debated criteria included age, sex, number of dependents, educational level, past performance and future potential, and the person's value to society. The debate was too painful for people to tolerate, so they found a simple solution. They decided to spend more money and produce more kidney machines.

Today the dollar requirements for such a solution are becoming astronomical, and the billions are not available. We could transfer billions from our defense budget and raise our health-spending percentage of GNP (gross national product) even higher. But that would only delay some of the ethical decision-making that faces all of us daily in the medical profession. Sooner or later we must face this issue squarely: How do we allocate our limited medical technology?

Standards of Social Justice

Ethicist Gene Outka outlines four standards of social justice as possible answers to the question of fair distribution of health care resources (*On Moral Medicine: Theological Perspectives in Medical Ethics,* ed. Stephen E. Lammers and Allen Verhey [William B. Eerdmans, 1987], pp. 633-43).

1. *To each according to merit or desert.* When deciding who should receive a limited medical care technology, one should look at the lifestyle of the patient. Outka writes:

> Consider the following bidders for emergency care: (1) a person with a heart attack who is seriously overweight; (2) a football hero who has suffered a concussion; (3) a man with lung cancer who has smoked cigarettes for forty years; (4) a 60-year-old man who has taken excellent care of himself and is suddenly stricken with leukemia; (5) a three year old girl who has swallowed poison left out carelessly by her parents; (6) a 14-year-old boy who has been beaten without provocation by a gang and suffers brain damage and recurrent attacks of uncontrollable terror; (7) a college student who has slashed his wrists (and not for the first time) from a psychological need for attention; (8) a women raised in the ghetto who is found unconscious due to an overdose of heroin.
>
> These cases help to show why the whole subject of medical treatment is so crucial and so perplexing.... People suffer in varying ratios the effects of their natural and undeserved vulnerabilities, the irresponsibility and brutality of others, and their own desires and weaknesses (pp. 634-35).

Another very relevant example is the treatment of AIDS contracted by a practicing homosexual. Many sicknesses are brought on by unhealthy lifestyles. Does that mean that the emergency room physician must make value judgments before deciding who gets the respirator? No, we must work at preventive measures in the society at large—anti-smoking, seat belts, weight-reduction diets—and treat every patient with compassion and forgiveness.

Some physicians make decisions after considering a patient's commitment to a future healthy lifestyle. A cardiologist told me that he will not refer a cardiac patient for heart bypass grafting (CABG) unless the patient agrees to stop smoking. There is good evidence that continuing smoking after the $15,000 CABG surgery nullifies the positive effects of the procedure after only two years.

From a Christian perspective, should one's religious beliefs and practices affect the decision when rationing health care? Should the non-Christian receive priority?

2. *To each according to societal contribution.* This standard gives priority to those who contribute most to the society at large. Here we must judge the social consequences of the patient's conduct—or the greatest good for the greatest number. This standard would exclude the young, the aged, and, in most cases, the poor. The Swedish Hospital "public committee" had difficulty applying this standard when deciding whose life to spare using the artificial kidney. Should the person who supports six children have preference over the unmarried artist? Is a teacher preferred over the drug dealer? What about the actor, the entertainer, the professional athlete, the television minister?

Decisions using this standard will vary from one society to another. In the United States, we might choose the younger person over the elderly, and the parent over the childless. In East Africa, the choices would be just the opposite. The elderly have many relationships that are severed at death; the young have few. The elderly carry the wisdom of the society and are highly respected. The childless patient should be saved to give that person the chance to have children. Children represent that stream of life that one receives from his parents and passes on to the next generation. Being childless is a tragedy from the African perspective.

Decisions using this standard will also vary from one generation to another. When I was in my residency training in the early 1970s, we did not admit anyone to the critical-care unit (CCU) who was older than sixty-five. Today the majority of CCU patients are well over sixty-five. What happened? Yesterday's CCU beds became today's intermediate-care beds, and today's CCU units are a showcase of expensive technology.

3. *To each according to need.* Here we run into the problem of distinguishing essential need from felt need or wants. A patient may request an expensive CAT (computerized axial tomography) scan of his head after suffering a headache of several days. He may need immediate reassurance that he does not have a brain tumor, but the

prudent doctor will recommend a less expensive approach. One person's medical needs may be far in excess of another's just because of the random nature of the occurrence of health crises. The needs of food and clothing and shelter are ever-present, but a health crisis may strike at random. Also, the threshold of recognizing one's needs varies among individuals. This week a 78-year-old woman came to my office after experiencing months of vaginal bleeding, which she interpreted not as an illness but as her "period returning again." Her cancer is now far beyond cure. Another woman experiencing the same symptoms would have seen me months ago.

The medical needs perceived by the sick in the third world are much different from the needs of people of the Western world working with them. When an American suffers from a headache, she may need two aspirin. When a Tanzanian suffers from a headache, he may need two chloroquine (for malaria). A well-to-do person may need admission to a hospital for eating the wrong thing. A destitute person may plead for admission just to receive one good meal.

4. *Similar treatment for similar cases.* This standard appeals to fairness and consistency. One class of people should not receive significantly different treatment from another because of income or geographic location. Everyone should have equal access to medical care. The collision comes when the goal of equal access meets the realities of finite resources. This standard would say that if a treatment for a particular rare, noncommunicable disease is inordinately expensive and the prospects for rehabilitation remote, then no one should receive that treatment and the funds should be made available to the many with other illnesses. There should be no distinction between the afflicted rich and the afflicted poor. Discrimination in the allocation of funds would be based on the categories of illnesses, not people.

Should similar treatment for similar cases apply only to those poor in our own country or to those poor throughout the world? Should a mission worker in Tanzania have his appendix removed in the mission hospital or should he fly to Nairobi for surgery under conditions of less risk?

The Problem of Wealth

Throughout the world the allocation of medical resources tends to follow the distribution of food. Ron Sider quotes Lester Brown:

> One reason it is possible for the world's affluent to ignore such tragedies [famine] is that changes have occurred in the way that famine manifests itself. In earlier historical periods . . . whole nations . . . experienced widespread starvation and death. Today the advancement in both national and international distribution systems has concentrated the effects of food scarcity among the world's poor, wherever they are (*Rich Christians in an Age of Hunger* [InterVarsity Press, 1977] p. 23).

This is also true concerning the access to health care. Throughout the world good health care is available to a society's powerful wealthy and denied to their powerless poor. In Tanzania the privileged fly to Europe for specialized care, depending upon their connections to power. A key factor in the allocation is "technical know-WHO"!

Who would not wish to see the best doctors and have the most promising treatments when hearing of impending death?

> Our fear of illness and dying may be so pronounced and immediate that we will seize the nearly automatic connections between privilege, wealth, and power if we can. We will do everything possible to have our kidney machines, even if the charts make it clear that many more would benefit from mandatory immunizations at a fraction of the cost (Outka, p. 641).

We can do more to improve the health of a country by improving its economy than by smothering the land with health care providers. Providing clean, easily accessible water supplies and safe sewage disposal will lead to a healthier population.

With increasing wealth, a society can reduce risks in all areas of life. A wealthy society can require that bridges and roads and automobiles meet certain safety standards. These rising standards become more expensive and lead to less risk taking as a society can afford them. This is true also in medical care. For instance, in the 1950s an excellent antibiotic was developed that cured a wide variety of infections, but it also killed one in ten thousand users. Americans decided that this was an unacceptable risk. So chloramphenicol is not used, except in specific life-threatening circumstances. Instead, doctors prescribe more expensive antibiotics. In Africa chloramphenicol is a widely used inexpensive treatment because the 1-to-10,000 risk of death is small compared with the many greater risks that threaten people every day. Does this mean that an American is worth more than an African?

Some Biblical Perspectives

How can the Bible instruct us about the allocation of our scarce medical resources? God makes no moral distinctions when dealing with people. God is not biased. God cares about the needs of persons on the fringes of society.

> *Matthew 5:45:* "He causes his sun to rise on the evil and the good, and sends rain on the righteous and unrighteous."
> *Deuteronomy 10:17-18:* "For the Lord your God ... shows no partiality and accepts no bribes. He defends the cause of the fatherless and the widow, and loves the alien, giving him food and clothing."

The early church was very concerned with meeting the needs of all (Acts 2:43-47; 4:32-37; 5:1-11; 6:1-7). Paul's letters reveal radically changed economic relationships among the people of God. Being "transformed by the renewing of your minds" (Romans 12:1-2) included an economic transformation. Paul's Second Letter to the Corinthians highlights the love gift that he was collecting from the Christians in Turkey and Greece for the poorer Christians in Jerusalem (2 Corinthians 8:13-15).

Is our situation any different today? More than half of our Christian brothers and sisters live outside of North America. Many are in the medically poor countries of the third world. If Paul were here today, would he not take an offering for the poor Christians in Tanzania, for example, where most families have lost at least one child to disease? Should we not provide at least minimal preventive care to the poorer of our body before we spend our resources selfishly on high-tech medical care? Can you imagine how the non-Christian world would react if they saw Christians selling their property to provide for the needs of their brothers and sisters in Christ?

Who Makes the Decisions?

1. *Patients or their families.* The decision to go for high tech or to refrain generally is made by the patient or the patient's family, usually in consultation with a physician. Other factors such as the insurance coverage, the availability of the service, and anticipated outcome are usually brought into consideration. But the final decision whether or not to "go for it" rests with the patient. Sometimes the decision results in an unpaid hospital bill which the hospital has to absorb and pass on to the paying patients.

2. *Private hospitals and emergency room physicians.* A private hospital may try to anticipate who are the nonpaying patients and transfer them to a government hospital, a practice called *dumping*. Patient dumping has increased by more than 500 percent in the Chicago area over the past few years. In 1985, 6,000 emergency patients were transferred to the Cook County Hospital, often when their medical condition was not stable enough for safe transport. (Daniel S. Greenberg, "If You're Poor, Don't Get Sick," *Chicago Tribune*, 29 July, 1985). In these cases, the decision for use of high tech was in the hands of the emergency room receiving physicians.

3. *Government (Medicare and Medicaid).* Through Medicare the federal government has restricted the use of an expensive medical resource—the hospital—through its DRG (diagnostic related groups) program, where the decision to pay for hospitalization days is based on the patient's diagnosis. Medicare patients with certain diagnoses, such as cataract, are not permitted to be hospitalized for their surgery. Yesterday I admitted a 98-year-old woman with two fractured vertebrae and broken ribs and was told that the hospital might reject the admission.

4. *Manufacturers of technology.* AZT (azidothymidine), the new drug for the treatment of AIDS, is controlled by the drug company. Doctors may apply for the expensive drug after supplying clinical data that indicate the severity of the patient's illness. A more severely ill patient will be granted the privilege of purchasing the drug—at a cost of $10,000 per year.

5. *Physicians.* Physicians differ in their approach to the use of technology. Some may be so convincing in their explanations that the patient or the family cannot refuse without feeling guilty. Some

may even initiate certain therapies without consulting anyone.

6. *Code-blue and emergency-medical-treatment teams.* A patient may be found in the hospital bed or in his backyard after suffering a cardiac arrest. The emergency team who come to his rescue may know nothing about the patient's medical history nor his wishes, and he receives thousands of dollars of technology before the appropriate decision-makers arrive on the scene.

7. *Third-party insurers.* Like the Medicare-Medicaid system, many insurance companies are trying to stem the rising tide of medical costs by limiting hospital admissions. All elective admissions must be approved in advance. All elective surgical procedures must be cleared by a second-opinion physician. After admitting a patient on an emergency basis, the patient's insurance company reviewer in some distant city calls the patient's physician and tells him or her the number of hospital days that the company will pay for.

What to Do?

1. *Petition government to allocate more medical services for the indigent.* During the past five years, medical care has turned into a commodity rather than a basic right for all people. Funding has been limited for the poor and the elderly. According to Lester A. Thurow, a three-tier system of medical care is unfolding:

> There will be a set of government health care providers who will provide the minimal level of health care for the poor and the elderly. . . . The level of health care will be determined by the per capita grant that the government is willing to pay. . . . The quality of the second tier will be established by private corporations and will depend on the level of health care that they are willing to provide for their employees. . . . The third tier will be a free-market, individual health care system. This will be the market in which people can buy health care in excess of that provided by their employers or the government. The only limit on treatment will be the amount of money that people are willing to spend on themselves or their family. ("Medicine versus Economics," *New England Journal of Medicine* 313:611-14.)

We must be more vocal in informing our government officials that we favor cuts in the military spending in favor of better health services for all, especially the poor and the elderly. We must expose excessive military budgets as demonic.

2. *Petition physicians to discuss the technology with you before making decisions about your care.* Discuss costs and the likelihood of benefit proportionate to the costs of the diagnostic test or treatment. Lester Thurow suggests further that "if one could convert all American doctors to the practice style of the group of competent doctors that uses each medical technique least, it would be possible to effect enormous savings without having to employ the unequal three-tiered health care system toward which we are now moving" (Thurow, p. 613).

3. *Discuss the use of high technology with your spouse or close friend so that you are better prepared to make decisions when the time arrives.* Will you want life-support systems to sustain you? Give someone power-of-attorney in case you lose your ability to make decisions. Then discuss these issues at length with that person so that he or she will be better able to participate in the agonizing decisions without guilt.

4. *Practice healthiness.* Discipline yourself toward weight control, blood-pressure control, stress reduction; and avoid drugs, cigarettes, and alcohol. Wear seat belts, get adequate sleep and exercise, check your cholesterol level, and have periodic health evaluations.

5. *Practice patience.* When an unusual symptom does arise, check with a knowledgeable health care provider and accept his or her advice. Then give the symptom some time to disappear before pushing for the expensive tests. Two of medicine's least expensive tests are time and reexamination.

6. *Consult your pastor.* Decisions about spending for high-tech medical services are moral and ethical decisions. Where are the pastors in this process? A caring physician should consult with you and your pastor and explain the risks, the costs, and the probable outcome of a particular technology. Unfortunately, there are so many unknowns, especially when deciding about cancer treatments, that probable outcome is often merely a guess. Yet a growing amount of data is becoming available on many of the high-tech modalities. Life-and-death decisions must be made within the community of faith. Perhaps a pastoral committee including health care providers within the fellowship could be helpful. However, if most of us are

reluctant to share our financial decisions with our sisters and brothers, will we be able to share our medical decisions?

A Modest Suggestion

Paul was so intent upon collecting money from the rich Christians in Asia Minor to help those poor Christians in Jerusalem that he put his life on the line in that effort. His goal was equality—"At the present time your plenty will supply what they need, so that in turn their plenty will supply what you need. Then there will be equality" (2 Corinthians 8:14). At the present time there is a disparity in the health care available within our Christian fellowships, even in North America. But the differences in health care available to North American and third world Christians are as vivid as white and black. What would Paul say about this inequality?

Why don't Christians in North America band together in a mutual attempt to care for all of our medical needs? All members of a denominational community could join and receive medical care with no exclusions for preexistent conditions. Each congregation would finance the plan according to the needs of the entire church during the past year. Those poorer churches would pay less per capita than the more wealthy churches. Those receiving medical benefits from their employers would request that their monthly benefit be transferred to a denominational health care plan. Standards of care should be established as basic, and discussions could begin to give guidelines as to when expensive high-tech procedures are used. Local committees would be actively involved in helping individuals and families in the church make health care decisions. There would be a "hotline" and phone consultations among denominational health care providers to assist those committees. At the end of a given year, congregations (or denominations) would send the money they saved to brothers and sisters with medical needs in North America and beyond our shores. Some denominational aid associations are already fulfilling some of these goals, but they could expand their work to facilitate this proposal.

This plan would allow Christians to become more responsible in health care matters. We might decide as congregations that certain high-tech procedures are not to be used as long as *our* children in the third world are dying of easily curable diseases.

Might some of our denominations become known as people who refuse high tech to provide for the welfare of their sisters and brothers? In the early church, when needs became apparent, love for the fellowship became a paramount concern. "No one claimed that any of his possessions was his own, but they shared everything they had" (Acts 4:32).

For Discussion

1. What standards should we use in deciding who gets expensive high-tech medical care, for example, liver transplants?

2. A 72-two-year-old patient with severe lung disease spent 120 days in the CCU on a respirator last year and eventually recovered from his illness. He is now living an independent lifestyle, although he is limited by shortness of breath and arthritis pains. Was it appropriate to spend $120,000 to treat this man? (The money came from Medicaid funds even though there may not be enough funds left for routine immunizations of the poor children in 1987.) Should the dollar sign be a factor in our decisions, since it means that less will be available for the many?

3. Are we as Christian communities exhibiting racism when we allow the disparity of health care to exist between our white and nonwhite members? Should we be willing to give up ownership of our possessions until there is not a needy person among us?

4. In 1986 there were approximately 30,000 cases of AIDS in the United States, with that number expected to double every fourteen months! Most AIDS victims are practicing homosexuals or drug abusers and will die a slow and costly death over a two-year period. How should we finance the care of these victims? How would you feel about paying more tax dollars for their care?

12

Prevention—and More!

Ann Raber

AFTER A CARDIOVASCULAR exam, Abraham Schmitt
learned that he needed bypass surgery. His identical twin received a
clean bill of health. Twelve years before, Abe's twin discovered that
his cholesterol reading was extremely high, so he took drastic re-
medial action. He switched to a low-sodium, low-cholesterol diet
and became a long-distance biker and jogger.

His twin's fanatic devotion to health turned Abe off. He
assumed that the physical activity of normal living was adequate.
As the years passed, his life became more and more sedentary as he
worked as an individual and marriage therapist in an office in his
house. And he banked on his good genealogy—to his knowledge
there had never been any heart disease in his family. But at age fifty-
eight, Abe had to pay the price for neglecting his heart.

After a quadruple heart bypass, regular exercise and a low-sodium, low-cholesterol diet became part of Abe's life. He cut out coffee completely. The change in eating habits was difficult, but the
rewards in improved health have been great.

Abe says, "If I could live the past sixteen years over again, I
would make drastic changes. First, I would stop fooling myself
about my naturally endowed gifts of good health and long life.

Next, I would reject the accepted American pattern of self-indulgence and leisure. Then I would learn about heart disease before I was forced into the crash course I have just completed. Finally, I would implement a program of appropriate regular systematic exercise and total dietary change. I would reduce any vocational stress with exercise, not more and more coffee."

■ ■ ■

God intends for us to live fully and abundantly, to live vibrantly. That kind of radiant living refers to the whole person—body, mind, and spirit. Health is so easy to ignore, at least until it isn't there. It's like the old story of being unaware of a big toe until a brick falls on it. Then suddenly that big toe becomes the focus of existence.

In the preceding chapters, we have studied several of the "big toe" issues of our time, such as organ transplants and genetic engineering. These are thorny problems with no simple solutions. Obviously, prevention would be preferable. Fortunately, in many cases prevention is a real possibility. We have learned a lot about the diseases that we face, and we know some things about preventing them.

We are living in the third phase of medical care in this culture. The first began in the late 1800s and extended well into the 1900s—a time of decreasing death rates and slowly improving environment. During this time the major killers were diseases such as diphtheria, smallpox, influenza—all infectious diseases. Major efforts in sanitation, public health, and education played primary roles in bringing those diseases under control. Some significant changes were the installation of running water in most homes, the purification of public water systems, and the general acceptance of improved personal hygiene as a routine practice. This was also the time in which we made major strides in science. The development and wide distribution of vaccines and antibiotics required scientific, educational, and governmental cooperation. So successful were these efforts—until the outbreak of AIDS in 1981—that infectious disease was well on the way to being controllable. In fact, some diseases that had earlier been significant causes of death, such as smallpox, were being talked about in the past tense.

During the 1940s the next phase began. This was the era of technology, of amazing surgery, and of almost miraculous achievements in the medical field. Procedures such as renal dialysis—drawing the blood out of someone's body, cleaning it, and then putting it back, and doing this over and over on a regular schedule—became routine. Only a few years ago this would have been totally unthinkable. The artificial heart is another splendid example of this technological phase. Joint replacements, artificial bionic limbs, and pacemakers are some others.

Exciting as these developments are, they are clearly a matter of much for a few. Most of us do not plan to live out our lives with a Jarvik heart. So while the capabilities are almost without limit, the actual impact on the life of the average person is minimal, except for the financial considerations. The health of the general public has not greatly improved because of these technological advances. In fact, during this period, death due to chronic disease began to develop as a serious concern. The cost of medical care went up dramatically, another negative development of these spectacular achievements.

We are in the third phase now. Beginning in the late 1960s, there has been a significant change in the major causes of death in this country. They are no longer the infectious diseases of that earlier era. Now they are the *lifestyle diseases*, those caused or greatly influenced by the way we live. They are the heart diseases, the cancers, accidents, and the alcohol- and other drug-related disorders. These diseases are associated with physically inactive lifestyles, diets containing too much fat, salt, and sugar, uncontrolled stress, lack of healthy self-respect, and a toxic environment.

There are no vaccinations for the lifestyle disorders. Our physicians cannot prevent them. These lifestyle disorders are the result of choices we make many times each day. The decisions we make, usually out of habit, affect the routine aspects of our lives in areas such as the following:

1. *Physical fitness.* We are designed for motion, but many of us lead such sedentary lives that our typical day involves very little motion. We know that many lifestyle diseases are related to a lack of exercise. We are now making the connection between physical

fitness and better performance on the job, better personal relations in the family, and better spiritual growth. Exercise is also one of the best methods of managing stress. It becomes clear that a well-functioning body makes it possible to function well in other areas too.

2. *Nutrition.* We are nearly overwhelmed by the flood of information coming from the research and the advertising in this area. We are learning how our eating habits affect our behavior and feelings. We read studies linking certain foods to cancer and heart disease. Many of us are still eating a diet traditional with farmers and other people doing lots of vigorous physical labor even though our lifestyles are largely sedentary. We tend to shop, cook, and order food on the basis of taste alone. Integrating nutrition into our Christian lifestyle will mean considering not only taste, but economy, ecology, and peace and justice issues as well.

3. *Stress management.* Stress is a part of life for each of us; and that's okay if we develop ways of handling it so that it does not damage us. Uncontrolled stress can cause a person to be irritable and unpleasant, as well as ill. However, a little stress can help us to be alert and vibrant, to thoroughly enjoy our work and service. Learning to manage stress does not always mean slowing down and doing nothing. It might mean doing more. We must learn to bring balance to our lives by controlling our responses to the events and pressures we encounter every day.

4. *Mental health.* Mental health encompasses a large part of who we are. It has to do with the vitality of our relationships, our intellectual curiosity, our joy in living, our openness to new ideas, our sense of humor, and our own self-respect.

By now you can see how each of these elements actually is a part of each of the others. In discussing one you inevitably wind up discussing another and another. That is one remarkable thing about wellness: by definition it equals *whole*.

5. *Spirituality.* The spiritual part of us that gives direction and purpose to our lives needs attention and nurturing just as our physical and emotional parts do. There is a wide resurgence of interest in spirituality, perhaps in response to the highly technical and impersonal nature of our age. But this is also an area that we don't understand very well. We are afraid of trying something unfamiliar for fear it might not be a path to God. Yet often we are not

experiencing much growth or satisfaction using the methods we have always used. So we remain stuck, never experiencing the joy and wonder that could be ours if we were committed to greater faithfulness and stewardship in our everyday lives.

Few of us will live a life of high drama that will be the epic told over and over for generations. However, the consistent, dedicated person that daily lives out the essence of her or his belief leaves a legacy of encouragement and strength, love, and inspiration, to all those around. That life of wellness speaks of God's will and plan for all God's people.

6. *The environment.* In Genesis 2, we read that God created the world and all the living things in it. God then turned this magnificent creation over to people to manage it. This precious earth is our responsibility, and we are now on the verge of seeing it totally destroyed. If we believe in a God of creation, we must take a serious look at how we are managing the world God gave us. This is part of our Christian stewardship. It is also part of keeping the world a healthy place for living beings to inhabit.

■ ■ ■

Being conscientious decision-makers in these areas will take us beyond prevention to wellness. John Travis says that most of us spend most of our lives being not really sick but not really well either. Wellness means much more than the absence of illness.

We are acquainted with the left side of the diagram on the following page. We have all known signs and symptoms such as fatigue, lack of energy, headaches, or frequent colds. Most of us have been ill and have gone to the doctor and been helped back to the neutral position. We have even known persons who have died prematurely, not because it was God's will, but because of many choices made over a long time.

Moving beyond the neutral point of no illness, we begin to look at what positive health or wellness might be. Think about what that would mean for you: more energy, a more flexible body, a more interesting spiritual life, lower cholesterol, closer relationships, more satisfaction in work, or greater appreciation of others. Wellness is much more than physical fitness.

Illness/Wellness Continuum

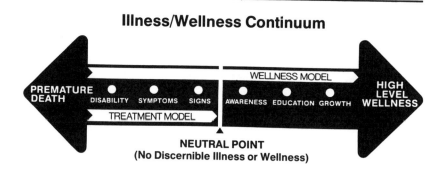

ILLNESS/WELLNESS CONTINUUM used with permission, Copyright 1972, 1981, John W. Travis M.D., Wellness Associates, Box 5433, Mill Valley, CA 94942. From *Wellness Workbook,* Ryan & Travis, Ten Speed Press, 1981

Actually, wellness has to do with living intentionally, not just doing what we have done habitually. Wellness means making deliberate choices and taking responsibility for those choices and their consequences. It means maintaining a balance between all the elements of myself so that no part is neglected or exaggerated. It means being a good steward of all that has been entrusted to me: my body, my time, my energy, my abilities, my resources. It means seeing myself and others as whole beings.

We need to accept our own role and power. We are responsible for what we eat, how we exercise, how we allow our stress to affect our lives and relationships, and how we schedule time to care for our spiritual development. At the same time, we need to be aware that we are not in control of everything. There are aspects of genetics, environment, pathology, for example, that we don't even understand, much less have power over. We need to be most humble about our own good health. We must be understanding and supportive of those not as fortunate as we. However, we should not use the fact that we don't control everything as an excuse not to control what we can.

Another of the elements that we can control is money. We can spend enormous amounts on spectacular treatments after years of unhealthy behavior. How often have we heard persons share their experiences of bypass surgery or severe heart attack and conclude by saying that now they feel better than ever. It's clear what happened—the person learned some significant lessons and made some wholesome changes. How much better it would be for us to learn without having a serious physical problem.

The question is not just one of dollars. As we saw in chapter 11, resources are limited and how we spend our money is one way in which we set forth our thinking and our priorities. If we are content to continue paying huge amounts of money for treatment while maintaining destructive personal habits, we send a distorted message to the world about our sense of Christian stewardship. We need to learn to care for each other in health-making ways, not in ways that contribute to ill health. We need to be more concerned for prevention and less for fantastic forms of treatment.

■ ■ ■

We come again to the idea of living intentionally rather than existing on "automatic pilot." It means seeing our Christian commitment as involving the details of how we live each day. We are discussing a healthy care of ourselves, so as to be able for God's work, to be fit for service. Our goal includes direction and purpose beyond ourselves, not the self-centered life that often is the result of a preoccupation with physical fitness. So what can we do?

When speaking to the Protestant Health and Welfare Assembly (1986), former governor of Colorado Richard Lamm said that government simply cannot afford the miracle cures and the fantastic technology. However, there are four elementary things that we could do that would make an immediate impact on the health of the nation and would improve the lives of millions at very little cost: (1) stop smoking, (2) eat wholesome foods, (3) control alcohol use, and (4) wear seat belts.

Robert Allen says that the habits we need to live longer and better are: be an intelligent eater, stay slim, don't smoke, don't drink heavily, get regular exercise, practice safety precautions, reduce stress, and have good mental health (Robert F. Allen and Shirley Linde, *Lifegain* [Norwalk, Conn.: Appleton-Century-Crofts, 1981], p. 14).

These are things that we all know we should do. Many of them we know how to do. Some of them we do. They are common sense. Maintaining the balance is the hard part. We tend to get carried away on one and ignore another.

We also want to put our whole lifestyle into the context of our Christian belief. Here are some simple—not necessarily easy—practical steps to take in moving toward prevention of disease and beyond to wellness.

First, accept personal responsibility. Believe that care of ourselves is part of God's plan, part of our stewardship requirement, part of God's quality control system. In doing that, we begin to take charge of our lifestyle.

Caring for ourselves is not a new concept. Most of the care of the sick has always been done by the patient, family, and friends. We have each made decisions about when to call the doctor, when to take an aspirin, or when to stay home in bed with a case of the flu. We are now moving to care for ourselves *before* we get sick, being smarter about living to eliminate some health risks.

That does not mean that we believe we can control everything. But it does mean that we understand that there are consequences related to all choices, and we are committed to making choices that produce the most positive results. The choices will probably require some change on our part. Going to the doctor for a checkup is good. However, it may be more important to begin an exercise program or a regular schedule of quiet time. As we begin making changes, small adaptations will be easier to make and easier to maintain than drastic ones. This way, over a period of time, we can make significant progress without enormous effort or disruption.

Second, we must accept our need to learn more about how we are living and what options are available to us. We will seek information on nutrition, exercise, and ways to enrich our spiritual lives. We will begin to be thoughtful about everyday matters that we did habitually and mindlessly before. We will begin to shop for health professionals who are concerned about our fitness as well as our illness. We will see ourselves as *partners* with our doctor, dentist, and others working for our well-being. We will ask more questions. We will experiment with new behaviors. We will listen to the signals that we get from our inner self.

For instance, how do you decide when to go to bed at night? When the news is over? Or when you're so exhausted that you simply cannot do another thing? Or is it with some consideration to the amount of sleep you need to be ready to meet a new day with energy and zest? Have you experimented with different amounts of sleep to determine what is best for you?

Do you know what your cholesterol level is? What it should be? How you can get it there? Do you know your resting heart rate? How you could lower it? What benefits might there be in lowering it? These are the kinds of questions that will come up as you begin to move toward a healthy lifestyle.

We must become smarter consumers. We have tended to believe what the advertisers have said. We have been readily seduced into buying products that are often worthless or even harmful. We must read labels and demand better information on ingredients. We must question those persons or systems that profit from our illness or lack of wellness. Food processors, tobacco companies, advertisers, even health care providers, may have a vested interest in our continuing destructive habits. It is our responsibility to ask the questions and make the choices that are good for us.

Third, we must accept our need for help. We cannot count on a lot of cultural support for making the lifestyle changes that move us toward positive health. Our culture is oriented toward watching sports on television, not participating in exercise. We tend toward filling each minute of every day with excitement and busyness, not scheduling time for reflection and quiet meditation. We are willing to accept prepackaged concepts, not discovering values and beliefs through thoughtful questioning and study. We need to build congregational support for the beliefs and practices that enable us to be well. And where, more than in the church, should we expect to find a community of persons willing to accept responsibility for themselves and each other, willing to see persons as whole, with all the complexities and differences—a true shalom community, living and experiencing total well-being?

We need the expertise of those with knowledge and training that we don't possess. We need their help, but we must stop expecting them to do everything for us. We need each other for support and accountability. We need each other to learn about ourselves.

Without others to question our beliefs and behaviors, we tend to assume the way we are is the only way to be. We need each other to develop a gentle sense of humor. Laughter is healthy. Norman Cousins calls it "internal jogging." To be able to see the absurd and laugh at ourselves is good stress management. It also helps us to keep things in perspective.

We need each other to learn about the beauty and vastness of God's creativity. The variety of shapes, sizes, colors, and styles of created beings reminds us to appreciate and celebrate differences, not be frightened by them. We need each other to work for change in our community life, to clean up the air, water, and soil, to work for peace and justice, to heal wounded relationships between persons, groups, and nations.

Each of us is in this world for a reason. We have work to do—and we do it better when we are well. Paul says, "Whether you eat or drink, or whatever you do, do all for the glory of God" (1 Corinthians 10:31). We have been talking about the "whatever," the everyday routines that enhance our lives and service or diminish the quality of our existence. The reward of wellness is more than the glory God receives. We also receive a more abundant life.

For Discussion

1. Read Matthew 22:37-39. How do we establish the Christian balance between caring for ourselves and caring for others?

2. How do we reconcile the abundant life to which we are called with the suffering that we are also taught to expect? What are the causes of suffering?

3. We have all received—which is the beginning of stewardship. What does being a good steward mean in terms of how we live? In decisions regarding prevention or treatment?

13

Where Do We Go from Here?

Erland Waltner

SEVERAL YEARS AGO, my mother, well into her ninety-first year, needed to be hospitalized because she could no longer swallow. Careful diagnostic tests turned up no clear medical problem, and the issue became whether to continue to force-feed her. The physician in charge sensitively outlined the problem and the options. The regimen of involuntary feeding, so obviously contrary to mother's desires, could prolong her life for weeks, months, or years. However, she would experience a minimal quality of life during a prolonged process of dying. As a family, we came to the painful consensus that we would not favor feeding mother against her will. So we had the feeding tube removed. However, instead of mother dying quickly, she began to rally and was given back to us for another eighteen months. At almost ninety-three, she died with dignity.

Father lived on several more years, blind but uncomplaining. He was ninety-seven when my brother telephoned to say that father was failing rapidly and that the nursing home attendants were asking whether we wanted him to return to the hospital, where more resuscitative technology would be available. Knowing that father could still communicate, I inquired whether they had asked him if he wanted to go to the hospital? His response to this option was an emphatic no. After checking with his physician and the nursing staff, we once again agreed to honor father's expressed preference. His death in the nursing home came very soon and mercifully.

The death of our beloved parents, both in Christian faith, included for us an experience we had not really anticipated. We were called on to participate in some ethical decisions concerning their health care in their final moments. Like so many others, we later asked, Did we do the right thing? We still think we did.

Responding to Medical Ethics

The preceding chapters have given us an introductory framework for thinking about and discussing from Christian perspectives some aspects of medical ethics. These have been identified by actual cases and by commentary. They have helped us understand something of the nature of the ethical dilemmas related to medical care, where several options may be possible and reasonable yet one has to choose. They have illustrated for us some of the deep complexities in the decision-making processes, some of which develop in critical moments and some of which stretch out over considerable time. They have indicated to us that life-and-death issues involve profound theological and ethical premises, which may be quite clear and explicit for some but which may be unexamined by others. They made us aware that the province of medical ethics in some sense belongs to the whole people of God, not only to health care professionals. They have nudged us in the direction of more congregational involvement in discussing these issues and in helping with ethical decision-making processes. They have given concrete handles to work on these matters.

We can respond in a number of ways. We may be quite overwhelmed by the difficulty and the complexity posed by the array of issues. Feeling bewildered, we may want to withdraw to the familiar posture of letting the health professionals decide—either the doctor "who knows best" or the medical ethics committees now available in some hospitals. However, as we have seen, the locus for decision-making is gradually being shifted and broadened beyond the professionals.

We may respond with some measure of anger, protesting that

surely the Bible must have clearer answers to all these questions than we have been given. We may feel that *someone* has let us down and that *someone* needs to get on the ball and figure out the right answers. This scapegoating will not work either, because for many of these issues there are no agreed-upon right answers.

Some very few of us may think that we have already learned so much about medical ethics that we may want to express our views on every ethical issue our friends are struggling with. The truth is that this book only scratches the surface. We must consider still more questions than have been raised here, and every new advance of medical technology tends to introduce still more.

Having experienced this introduction, now we may want to go on to learn still more, to understand better, and to begin to identify and appropriate personally, congregationally, and institutionally the implications of what we have learned. In short, we really want to learn how to discern between what leads to life and what leads to death in the more than physical sense of both terms.

In any case, we should see this book as a sign pointing the way toward further exploration and not as an answer book to difficult ethical questions.

Some Emerging Postures

Written by a variety of persons representing various disciplines and different experiences, it is noteworthy that some broad lines of agreement do emerge. In the case of these chapters, all writers begin with premises arising out of Christian faith, which is not the case when one examines the larger body of literature on medical ethics. Some approaches to life do not assume a Christian view of person, of life beyond human death, or of one who is Lord over life and death (Romans 14:9).

Basically, the writers agree that ethical decision-making is complex and cannot be satisfied with glib answers. The approach is humility and searching rather than proclamation and pontification.

They agree that the advance of medical technology is a major factor in the current dilemmas. They do not bemoan these advances as tragedy but recognize them as given reality. No one whines for some "good old days" before the benefits of modern medical technology were available.

They also agree that in the use of medical technology we encounter a major cost factor. High tech generally means high cost. This appears to be a growing problem rather than one that is becoming more manageable. Once the doctor could say firmly, "We have done all we can do." Now, with vastly enlarged medical knowledge and technical resources, the doctor can rarely speak in such final terms. This, in turn, leads to inflated expectations from patients and their families. Perceived medical possibilities are translated into "infinite need." However, medical resources remain finite, though not fixed. Thus the stewardship of medical technology becomes a critical issue.

The writers identify the issue of *Who decides?* as fundamental. For a time, the physician in charge was the ultimate decision-maker. He or she received this power from the patient, the family, the insurance company, and society very broadly. Gradually this is changing, especially in that the personhood of the patient is being rediscovered. And since the patient exists in the context of family and society, medical ethics becomes more than a private negotiation between physician and patient. This immediately makes the decision-making process more complex.

The writers agree that the church has a role to play at various levels in responding to ethical dilemmas in relation to medical care. At a theological level, much more help is needed in discerning the biblical-ethical grounds for decisions. Very few of the many books written on medical ethics explore in depth the place and significance of the Bible in this process.

They also agree that congregations ought to become involved in discussion of medical ethics so that persons will be better prepared to face such issues themselves and to be more supportive to other persons in the congregation who are struggling. "If one part suffers, every part suffers with it" (1 Corinthians 12:26a).

The writers indicate that in some ways the medical focus is shifting from preoccupation with treatment and cure to prevention, from centering on illness to centering on wellness. This shift has far-reaching implications for all people, not just medical professionals. This is an area in which congregations can play a very significant role in education and motivation.

Additional Agenda

Medical ethics is larger than the range of issues covered by the preceding chapters. A helpful, though significantly more technical, anthology that gives a broader picture is *On Moral Medicine: Theological Perspectives in Medical Ethics*, edited by Lammers and Verhey (see bibliography). Additional areas of concern and exploration include:

1. The relationship between religion and medicine, and between theology and medical ethics.

2. The specific implications of your religious tradition or heritage for the practice of medical ethics.

3. The ethics of medical professionals in their relationships to each other, to their patients, and to society.

4. The ethics of prayer and faith healing; the boundary between faith claims and fraud.

5. The ethics of patient care, responding to the less obvious forms of pain and impoverishment.

6. The ethics of contraception and abortion, including the issue of when human life begins and what kinds of rights this implies.

7. The ethics of various types of psychiatric treatment—chemical, analytic, and surgical.

8. The ethics of medical ministry to the disabled.

9. The ethics of medical experimentation using animal and human subjects to increase medical knowledge.

10. The ethics of medical entrepreneurship and various kinds of socialized medicine.

11. The ethics of medical insurance, malpractice insurance, and malpractice lawsuits brought by patients and their families.

12. The response to persons with Acquired Immune Deficiency Syndrome (AIDS), including both health care and implications for lifestyle.

Possible Next Steps

1. This massive field calls for a new kind of biblical-ethical scholar who is competently conversant with the field of scientific medicine and competent in biblical-ethical studies. We will need a

cadre of scholars who can provide further leadership in carrying forward such discussions as have been introduced above. Such persons might already be involved in biblical-ethical studies but now need to become more competent in the basics of scientific medicine. On the other hand, persons involved in the practice or teaching of medicine now may need to enter more deeply into formal biblical-ethical studies.

2. We need to develop settings and processes for discussing some of the issues identified in this book. Leadership in such discussions, whether in church-school classes or special-interest groups, may well be shared by medical professionals (physicians, nurses, clinic or hospital staff, etc.) and pastors, pastoral counselors, chaplains, or other theologically oriented persons. This book may serve as an introductory text; but many other resources, some of which appear in the bibliography, can be pursued fruitfully. Such discussions must provide ample opportunity for participants to express their own questions, anxieties, hopes, and intentions. Such group experiences should aim to inform, to motivate, and (where appropriate) to implement action.

3. We may need to give more attention in our Bible schools, colleges, and seminaries to equipping future church leaders more adequately for their ministries in the areas of ethical discernment and decision-making in relation to medical concerns. Already some institutions are giving special attention to this. But since the call is to provide leadership to congregations in this area, something more than now prevails needs to emerge.

Likewise, those who are already in church leadership will need to have these matters introduced in pastors' workshops and seminars, continuing-education programs, and supervised reading courses. Church leaders need to catch a vision of the need and develop awareness of resources in terms of personnel and literature available for medical-ethics discussion groups, which may be set up either on a congregational, institutional, or community level.

4. Additional special forums with interdisciplinary participation ought to be planned at conference and institutional levels to probe much more deeply these profound issues: What is life? What is death? What is health? What is illness? What is healing? What is deliverance? What is humanness and what are its boundaries? These

questions need to be looked at again, not only in the presence of the medical ethics issues that have been raised, but also from the perspective of the biblical meaning of shalom, salvation, discipleship, and caring community. Eventually such forums should lead to a clarified methodology as to how physician and pastor, their medical teams and their pastoral associates, can work together in health concerns and in medical ethics decision-making to help people respond to life-and-death issues with hope, courage, and joy rather than timidity and anxiety.

5. A reexamination of our worship and preaching patterns in the life of local congregations may also be called for. Granger West- berg has suggested that the Sunday morning worship ought to be a congregation's healthiest moment of the week. But if that is to be- come true, we may need to ask how healthy and healing our wor- ship services really are. Do our congregational worship and our preaching ministries help people to choose between life and death in the fullest sense? Do they motivate persons to move toward God's intended health and wholeness for their lives? Are we enabling broken, distressed, or diseased persons facing the realities of life and death to commune with the one who is our ultimate health and sal- vation?

6. We will want to examine our congregational curriculum and other educational activities to see what place life-and-death issues currently have in what our children, youth, and younger and older adults are studying. Because the issues of life and death go to the very core of our existence, it will not be satisfactory to leave educa- tion in ethical issues to our public schools. While we can appreciate and support much that our public schools may be doing within the boundaries of a pluralistic society, it will no longer do to have our children learn about sex and AIDS in the public arena only. Neither are Christian parents alone generally able to handle such volatile issues in their homes. Here the congregation, through a network of informed and concerned parents, has an opportunity to lay solid foundations for ethical living and decision-making.

7. Many congregations may see the need for setting up a con- gregational health concerns council. Such a council can become the local coordinating agency for health education, promoting dis- cussions on medical ethics, ministries to the aging, ministries to the

disabled and their families, or for any group or activity where health or wellness becomes a focal concern.

Where Do We Go from Here?

Personally, we can begin at once to face our own health needs and to strengthen a lifestyle of wellness along the lines outlined by Ann Raber in chapter 12. We can get in touch with our own aging process, begin to see life more holistically, and seek to make the right choices for life in all of its fullness as God intended (John 10:10).

Congregationally, we can begin modestly to help our people become aware of the issues and the resources available to work through those issues. We may encourage our church leaders to bring into being the kind of settings and structures that will make continuing discussion of medical ethics issues possible and fruitful.

Institutionally, depending on what type of institutions we are part of, we will examine ourselves to see in what ways our purposes are congruent with a Christian approach to life-and-death issues and to establish structures and processes that can be responsive.

God is surely manifest and active in the Christian concern to find a way through current medical ethics issues. This is obviously not the only item on the agenda for the church today. Yet because it is so deeply personal and paramount, because it is so relevant to all segments of congregational life, and because it is so inextricably bound up with the meaning and implications of the biblical gospel—for these reasons, we may hope that our wrestling with medical ethics under the power and control of the Holy Spirit will help to renew our theology and ethics and our experience of God's life-giving and healing presence among us as the people of God.

Let us allow God's Spirit to inspire us concerning the next steps we may take individually, congregationally, and institutionally. Let us learn to pray about these matters and allow God to begin to act out life rather than death in us and through us.

For Discussion

1. Encourage group members to express their feeling response to this book as a whole. What has been most helpful? Why?

2. Reviewing the list of items that have not been probed deeply

in this book, which additional items should have priority in further study? Why?

3. Review suggestions for next steps. At what point do you feel led to begin personally? How can you be helpful to some other person and to your congregation now that you have worked through this book?

Appendix

Ways to Lead a Group Study Using This Book

John Rogers

MENNONITE MUTUAL AID commissioned this book to help people in congregations to (1) begin to understand how to apply their Christian faith to areas of medical crisis that fellow members face, (2) become knowledgeable and sensitive caregivers at times of medical crisis, and (3) be able to interact with the medical-health care system with strength and authority rather than with fear and timidity. So if you are reading and studying this book within a congregational grouping—a small group, a Sunday school class, a pastoral-care team—here are a few points to keep in mind.

Chapters 1-7 identify and discuss broad principles that we should consider when facing medical crises. They provide helpful background for other chapters that deal with specific crisis situations. It is possible to read, understand, discuss, and apply the information in chapters 8-13 without having read chapters 1-7. But being aware of the principles presented there would enhance your study of specific concerns.

If you are reading and studying this book as part of a small group or a pastoral-care team and want to give most of your time to chapters 8-13, individuals could read chapters 1-7 as background. You might have someone provide a written summary of the principles in those chapters and begin your study by discussing this summary. Then the group could start studying specific issues.

If you are reading and studying this book as a Sunday school class, you might find it difficult to stay with the book for thirteen consecutive weeks. So you might want to read and study the book in two parts—chapters 1-7 and chapters 8-13—with a break in between. The potential problem with this approach is that people may want to focus only on specific issues without discussing the principles. If the class feels strongly about this, you can go directly to chapters 8-13, but be sure to encourage people to read chapters 1-7 on their own. Another option is to ask two or three people to commit themselves to read these chapters and to continually relate what they learn to the specific issues the class is discussing. Or you might have these persons share their learning in the first class of the study—perhaps in writing.

The questions at the end of each chapter are designed to help persons deal with the issues in the chapter at a personal level. The goal is to acquire information and to get in touch with feelings and beliefs. You might find it helpful to begin each class by discussing one of the questions at the end of the chapter to get people personally involved. Then you could review the content of the chapter, being sure to give time for persons to raise concerns or issues or to ask their own questions. Finally, conclude by discussing the remaining questions at the end of the chapter.

Regardless of what type of group you are part of, one aim is to enhance your congregation's ability to care for persons in medical crises. So you might want to keep this aim in mind throughout your study and present a summary of your group's learning to the appropriate person(s)—for example, the pastor or the pastoral-care team—when you finish. It is better to work at this summary throughout the course of the study rather than waiting until you have finished. To do this, here are questions that you might ask at the end of each session:

1. What are the key issues that this chapter raises for us as a congregation?

2. What strengths and weaknesses does this chapter point up in our congregational caring?

3. What remedies does the chapter suggest? What other

remedies might we consider?

4. How might we begin to implement these remedies in our congregation?

When you have finished the study, compare the answers to these questions for each chapter. Identify the responses that appear repeatedly. Establish a priority among these responses as a guide for working at improving your congregation's caring ministry. Finally, share the result of your study with the appropriate person(s) in your congregation.

Bibliography

Allen, David E., Lewis P. Bird, and Robert Herrmann, eds. *Whole-Person Medicine: An International Symposium.* Downers Grove, Ill.: Inter-Varsity Press, 1980.

Ashley, Benedict M., and Kevin D. O'Rourke. *Health Care Ethics: A Theological Analysis.* 2d ed. St. Louis: Catholic Health Association of the United States, 1982.

Bailey, Lloyd R., Sr. *Biblical Perspectives on Death.* Overtures to Biblical Theology. Philadelphia: Fortress Press, 1979.

Bakken, Kenneth L. *The Call to Wholeness: Health as a Spiritual Journey.* New York: Crossroad Publishing Co., 1985.

Beauchamp, Tom L. and James F. Childress. *Principles of Biomedical Ethics.* 2d. ed. New York: Oxford University Press, 1983.

Bender, David L., ed. *Death and Dying: Opposing Viewpoints.* 2d. rev. ed. St. Paul: Greenhaven Press, 1987.

Born Dying. 16mm film and ¾" videocassette, 20 min. Urbana, Ill.: Carle Medical Communications.

Childress, James F. *Priorities in Biomedical Ethics.* Philadelphia: Westminster Press, 1981.

_____. *Who Should Decide? Paternalism in Health Care.* New York: Oxford University Press, 1982.

Doss, Richard W. *The Last Enemy: A Christian Understanding of Death.* San Francisco: Harper and Row, 1974.

Feifel, Herman, ed. *New Meanings of Death.* New York: McGraw-Hill Book Co., 1977.

Gustafson, James M. *The Contributions of Theology to Medical Ethics.* Milwaukee: Marquette University Press, 1975.

Harron, Frank. *Human Values in Medicine and Health Care: Audio-Visual Resources.* New Haven: Yale University Press, 1983.

Harron, Frank, John Burnside, and Tom Beauchamp. *Health and Human Values: A Guide to Making Your Own Decisions.* New Haven: Yale University Press, 1983.

Hauerwas, Stanley. *A Community of Character: Toward a Constructive Christian Social Ethic.* Notre Dame, Ind.: University of Notre Dame Press, 1981.

_____. *Suffering Presence: Theological Reflections on Medicine, the Mentally Handicapped, and the Church.* Notre Dame, Ind.: University of Notre Dame Press, 1986.

Huttman, Barbara. *The Patient's Advocate.* New York: Viking Press, 1981.

Janzen, Waldemar. *Still in the Image: Essays in Biblical Theology and Anthropology.* Newton, Kans.: Faith and Life Press, 1982.

Jones, D. Gareth. *Brave New People: Ethical Issues at the Commencement of Life.* Rev. ed. Grand Rapids: William B. Eerdmans Publishing Co., 1985.

Kung, Hans. *Eternal Life? Life After Death as a Medical, Philosophical, and Theological Problem.* Translated by Edward Quinn. New York: Doubleday and Co., 1984.

Lammers, Stephen E., and Allen Verhey, eds. *On Moral Medicine: Theological Perspectives in Medical Ethics.* Grand Rapids: William B. Eerdmans Publishing Co., 1987.

Marty, Martin E., and Kenneth L. Vaux. *Health, Medicine and the Faith Traditions: An Inquiry into Religion and Medicine.* Philadelphia: Fortress Press, 1982.

May, William F. *The Physician's Covenant: Images of the Healer in Medical Ethics.* Philadelphia: Westminster Press, 1983.

Naisbitt, John. *Megatrends: Ten New Directions Transforming Our Lives.* New York: Warner Books, Inc., 1982.

No Heroic Measures. 16mm film and ¾″ videocassette, 23 minutes. Urbana, Ill.: Carle Medical Communications.

O'Rourke, Kevin, and Dennis Brodeur. *Medical Ethics: Common Ground for Understanding.* St. Louis: Catholic Health Association of the United States, 1986.

Payne, Franklin E., Jr. *Biblical/Medical Ethics: The Christian and the Practice of Medicine.* Milford, Mich: Mott Media, Inc., 1985.

President's Commission for the Study of Ethical Problems in Medicine and Biomedical and Behavioral Research. *Deciding to Forego Life-Sustaining Treatment.* Washington, D.C.: U.S. Government Printing Office, 1983.

_____. *Making Health Care Decisions: Informed Consent.* Washington, D.C.: U.S. Government Printing Office, 1982.

Ramsey, Paul. *Ethics at the Edges of Life: Medical and Legal Intersections.* New Haven: Yale University Press, 1978.

Reiser, Stanley Joel, Arthur J. Dyck, and William J. Curran, eds. *Ethics in Medicine: Historical Perspectives and Contemporary Concerns.* Cambridge, Mass.: MIT Press, 1977.

Robertson, John A. "Surrogate Mothers: Not So Novel After All." *The Hastings Center Report* (October 1983): 29-34.

Rogers, John, and Mary Ellen Martin, eds. *A Life of Wholeness: Reflections on Abundant Living.* Scottdale, Pa.: Mennonite Publishing House, 1983.

Schneider, Edward D., ed. *Questions About the Beginning of Life: Christian Appraisals of Seven Bioethical Issues.* Minneapolis: Augsburg Publishing House, 1985.

Sehnert, Keith W. *SelfCare/WellCare: What You Can Do to Live a Healthy, Happy, Longer Life.* Minneapolis: Augsburg Publishing House, 1985.

Seybold, Klaus, and Ulrich B. Mueller. *Sickness and Healing.* Translated by Douglas W. Stott. Nashville: Abingdon Press, 1981.

Shelly, Judith Allen. *Dilemma: A Nurse's Guide for Making Ethical Decisions.* Downers Grove, Ill.: Inter-Varsity Press, 1980.

Siegler, Miriam, and Humphry Osmond. *Patienthood: The Art of Being a Responsible Patient.* New York: Macmillan Publishing Co., 1979.

Simmons, Paul D. *Birth and Death: Bioethical Decision-Making.* Biblical Perspectives on Current Issues. Philadelphia: Westminster Press, 1983.

Singer, Peter, and Helga Kuhse. *Should the Baby Live?* New York: Oxford University Press, 1985.

Tournier, Paul. *The Whole Person in a Broken World: A Biblical Remedy for Today's World.* San Francisco: Harper and Row, 1981.

Tubesing, Donald A., and Nancy Loving Tubesing. *The Caring Question: You First Or Me First—Choosing a Healthy Balance.* Minneapolis: Augsburg Publishing House, 1983.

Veatch, Robert M. *Death, Dying, and the Biological Revolution: Our Last*

Quest for Responsibility. New Haven: Yale University Press, 1976.

Veatch, Robert M. *A Theory of Medical Ethics.* New York: Basic Books, 1981.

Westberg, Granger E., ed. *Theological Roots of Wholistic Health Care.* Hinsdale, Ill.: Wholistic Health Centers, 1979.

Westermann, Claus. *Creation.* Translated by John J. Scullion. Philadelphia: Fortress Press, 1974.

White, Dale, ed. *Dialogue in Medicine and Theology.* Nashville: Abingdon Press, 1968.

Winslade, William and Judith Ross. *Choosing Life or Death: A Guide for Patients, Families, and Professionals.* New York: Free Press, 1986.

Wright, Richard A. *Human Values in Health Care: The Practice of Ethics.* New York: McGraw-Hill Book Co., 1987.